CONTENTS

STATEMENTS

WEDNESDAY, APRIL 29, 1998

S. HRG. 105–518

ASSISTIVE TECHNOLOGY

HEARING

OF THE

COMMITTEE ON LABOR AND HUMAN RESOURCES UNITED STATES SENATE

ONE HUNDRED FIFTH CONGRESS

SECOND SESSION

ON

EXAMINING HOW ASSISTIVE TECHNOLOGY SHOULD BE DEVELOPED INTO THE 21ST CENTURY TO ADEQUATELY MEET THE NEEDS OF PERSONS WITH DISABILITIES, FOCUSING ON PROPOSED LEGISLATION TO AUTHORIZE FUNDS FOR PROGRAMS OF THE TECHNOLOGY-RELATED ASSISTANCE FOR INDIVIDUALS WITH DISABILITIES ACT OF 1988 (PUBLIC LAW 100–407)

APRIL 29, 1998

Printed for the use of the Committee on Labor and Human Resources

U.S. GOVERNMENT PRINTING OFFICE

48–228 CC WASHINGTON : 1998

For sale by the U.S. Government Printing Office
Superintendent of Documents, Congressional Sales Office, Washington, DC 20402
ISBN 0-16-057158-8

COMMITTEE ON LABOR AND HUMAN RESOURCES

JAMES M. JEFFORDS, Vermont, *Chairman*

DAN COATS, Indiana	EDWARD M. KENNEDY, Massachusetts
JUDD GREGG, New Hampshire	CHRISTOPHER J. DODD, Connecticut
BILL FRIST, Tennessee	TOM HARKIN, Iowa
MIKE DeWINE, Ohio	BARBARA A. MIKULSKI, Maryland
MICHAEL B. ENZI, Wyoming	JEFF BINGAMAN, New Mexico
TIM HUTCHINSON, Arkansas	PAUL D. WELLSTONE, Minnesota
SUSAN M. COLLINS, Maine	PATTY MURRAY, Washington
JOHN W. WARNER, Virginia	JACK REED, Rhode Island
MITCH McCONNELL, Kentucky	

MARK E. POWDEN, *Staff Director*
SUSAN K. HATTAN, *Deputy Staff Director*
WILLIAM G. DAUSTER, *Minority Chief of Staff and Chief Counsel*

ASSISTIVE TECHNOLOGY

WEDNESDAY, APRIL 29, 1998

U.S. SENATE,
COMMITTEE ON LABOR AND HUMAN RESOURCES,
Washington, DC.

The committee met, pursuant to notice, at 10:02 a.m., in room SD–430, Dirksen Senate Office Building, Senator Jeffords (chairman of the committee) presiding.

Present: Senators Jeffords, Frist, Hutchinson, Harkin, Wellstone, and Murray.

OPENING STATEMENT OF SENATOR JEFFORDS

The CHAIRMAN. The Committee on Labor and Human Resources will come to order.

This hearing on assistive technology will come to order, and I must say that the enthusiasm that I see among those who have turned out and those who are waiting outside reassures me in the knowledge that what has been going on has been helpful and productive in this area. It has been some 10 years since the first bill in this area was passed.

I would like to point out that we have both oral and sign interpreters available to assist individuals with testimony and questioning. Would the interpreters who sign please raise their hands? Thank you.

Would the oral interpreters please identify themselves? Thank you very much.

Now, anyone who would like to rearrange his or her seating in order to have a clear view of the interpreter under those circumstances, please do so now.

I would also like to say that I invited Senator Bond to testify today because of his interest in increasing R and D funding in assistive technology as well as funding Title III of the Tech Act on the Micro Loan Program. Unfortunately, his schedule did not allow him to be here today, but he is submitting a statement for the record, and I am sure he will be a strong supporter of assistive technology throughout the legislative process as he has been in the past. So I commend him for the work he has done in this area.

[The prepared statement of Senator Bond follows:]

PREPARED STATEMENT OF SENATOR CHRISTOPHER S. BOND

I thank the distinguished Chairman for giving me the opportunity to speak before the Committee on Labor and Human Resources about assistive technology, an issue that affects more than 15.6 million users and potential users of assistive technology in America.

Assistive technology provides a disabled individual the means to function better in the workplace or the home. This technology, which aids millions of Americans with physical or mental disabilities, improves the end users' quality of life as well as renders a means for acquiring a job. For example, assistive technology is a computer that can be used by an individual with Cerebral Palsy, a motor scooter or hearing aid for an individual who is aging, or enhanced voice recognition for someone with Multiple Sclerosis. Purchasing, gaining access and information to assistive technology, and many other problems are significant challenges for disabled persons, their families, guardians, or partners.

There is much work that needs to be done in the area of assistive technology on the Federal level—which will address these concerns and help state, local, private and nonprofit endeavors.

My staff and I have met with and contacted many agencies, organizations, and individuals involved in assistive technology research and development, information dissemination, training, education, funding and service delivery, such as the Department of Education's National Institute on Disability Research and Rehabilitation, the National Institutes of Health, the National Science Foundation, the Small Business Administration, the National Institute on Aging, the Federal Laboratory Consortium, the Social Security Administration and the National Council on Disability; as well as numerous advocacy groups including United Cerebral Palsy, NCD's Tech Watch program, Rehabilitation Engineering and Assistive Technology Society of North America, Brain Injury Institute, Friends of NIDRR, National Easter Seals, President's Committee on Employment of People with Disabilities, National Association of Protection and Advocacy Systems, Association of Tech Act Projects, American Foundation for the Blind, National Federation of the Blind. Also, we met with several Tech Act Project Directors including Missouri, Virginia, Iowa, North Carolina, and New York. Most importantly, we have sought the advice of those individuals who are most impacted by assistive technology—the end users. Their advice has been instrumental in the development of legislation that I intend to introduce soon.

I list all of these groups and individuals to illustrate the complex nature of this issue and the widespread impact that assistive technology has on the communities throughout America. Although this is a good representation of those involved in assistive technology, it is by no means exhaustive. Again, however, it is important to note the scope and depth of this issue which has driven me thus far in my search to find a perfect solution to the problems facing the assistive technology community.

As many of these groups expressed and as I have fully realized, there is no perfect solution. There are major problems existing in the assistive technology area which include a lack of awareness, service delivery, funding, and coordination of assistive technology research and development. A study by the Institute of Medicine entitled Enabling America: Assessing the Role of Rehabilitation Science and Engineering, which I based an initial draft of legislation, highlights many of these existing problems. However, as I have observed, many groups and individuals have major concerns about IOMs proposal.

The IOM study recommends three options to revise current federal assistive technology policy: improve the role of NIDRR; consolidate all federal programs involved in assistive technology research and development into a new agency; or create a new agency at the Department of Health and Human Services.

After a round table discussion in Missouri and a national round table discussion last week with the disability community, it is clear that the IOM's recommendation for improving the role of NIDRR is the principal choice to improve the Federal Government's role in assistive technology. Thus, Congress must act soon to improve NIDRR's role at the Department of Education, increase it's authority and improve its peer review process. It is my goal to make these areas the focus of new legislation, as well as including tax incentives for purchasing assistive technology for employees with disabilities and increased small business investment programs.

Most people with disabilities rely on assistive technology. In my home State of Missouri, the Assistive Technology Project focuses on assistive technology across ages, disabilities, and funding systems. The Missouri project has had much success including: establishing a low interest loan program with a statewide commercial bank to assist Missourians with disabilities in borrowing money to purchase this technology; securing private dollars to help support a statewide assistive technology conference and other training events; developing a statewide equipment recycling program to support the purchase, trade or give away of "pre-owned" assistive technology; and establishing regional assistive technology outreach centers that provide individual support to over 3,000 consumers annually and another 10,000 annually with assistive technology information.

To ensure the continuation of these successes, the Tech Act must be reauthorized. The State Tech Act projects are the lifeblood to the end users of assistive technology and their families, friends, and employers. The existing structure must be maintained to support current critical activities with a few modifications. All States and territories must receive a full 10-year funding cycle and Federal support must be provided beyond the 10-year cycle to address emerging and on-going assistive technology needs. Goals of legislation must enhance the ability of the State Tech Act projects to better coordinate, improve training and information dissemination, increase career enhancement/obtainment programs through assistive technology acquisition, and demand accountability. Finally, I will work to provide funding for Title III of the Tech Act's alternative financing mechanism's micro loan program.

Again, I thank the Chair, and I look forward to working with the committee to assure a bipartisan re-authorization of the State Tech Act Projects. Although there may not be a perfect solution for the problems facing the assistive technology community, I will work tirelessly with the Labor Committee to create legislation that will improve the lives of the millions of Americans with disabling conditions.

The CHAIRMAN. There is no doubt that we live in an information age. Information is power; it frees us. With information, each of us has the power to learn and to understand, to choose and to act. For all individuals, but especially those with disabilities, technology is the bridge to information, to choices and to freedom.

Ten years ago this month, Senator Harkin and I embarked on a joint venture. He in the Senate and I in the House decided to write legislation—the Technology-Related Assistance for Individuals with Disabilities Act of 1988. It has been known as the Tech Act.

We believed that technology was going to change our lives, change our expectations of ourselves and of each other. We wanted to make sure that the evolution, perhaps the revolution, in front of us included people wit disabilities. The Tech Act was our answer.

Within 6 months, we drafted legislation and then passed it on the same day in both Houses of Congress. It was signed into law by President Bush in August and received an appropriation that September.

The Tech Act authorized Federal funding for State grants to create tech projects. Tech projects then and now have served as catalysts to change Sate laws and policy related to assistive technology, to increase awareness of assistive technology and to promote increased access to it among individuals with disabilities.

We need to build the same momentum today that we had in 1988. In 1998, technology has become an integral part of our everyday life—at home, at school, at work and a play. Assistive technology plays a greater role in American life than most of us realize. For example, I wear a hearing aid as an assistive technology device. Rapid advances in information technology, the shift to managed care and its impact on insurance coverage of technology, and other issues present many new challenges in the assistive technology arena. We cannot allow these challenges to become barriers to accessibility.

I am looking forward to the testimony that we will hear today and to the expo on assistive technology that the Rehabilitation Engineering and Assistive Technology Society of North America has helped us organize for this afternoon. I think you will find it an incredible exhibit. Witnesses this morning and the exhibitors this afternoon will demonstrate how assistive technology has changed lives and dreams. They will demonstrate the power of partnerships and the importance of coordination. They will remind us that there continue to be roles for Federal and State governments, services providers, corporate America and, most importantly, individuals with disabilities and their families, in shaping America's investment in assistive technology.

The concern that my friend Tom Harkin and I shared in 1988 is still valid. Without access to the latest advances in technology, individuals with disabilities will be left behind. With access technology, they will walk the walk, talk the talk and dream the dreams that know no boundaries. We should settle for no less.

It is a pleasure to have as our first witness our good friend, Secretary Judith Heumann. We welcome you once again. Ms. Heumann is Assistant Secretary for the Office of Special Education and Rehabilitative Services. I think you must be approaching a record for the number of times you have testified in front of this committee, and each time, you do a stellar job. I look forward to your testimony.

Please proceed.

STATEMENT OF JUDITH E. HEUMANN, ASSISTANT SECRETARY, OFFICE OF SPECIAL EDUCATION AND REHABILITATIVE SERVICES, U.S. DEPARTMENT OF EDUCATION, WASHINGTON, DC, ACCOMPANIED BY KATHERINE D. SEELMAN, DIRECTOR, NATIONAL INSTITUTE ON DISABILITY AND REHABILITATION RESEARCH, AND CAROL CICHOWSKI, BUDGET OFFICE, U.S. DEPARTMENT OF EDUCATION

Ms. HEUMANN. Thank you, Mr. Chairman.

May I first introduce the people at the table with me. To me left is Kate Seelman, who is the director of the National Institute on Disability and Rehabilitation Research, which is a part of OSERS; and to my right is Carol Cichowski from the Budget Office in the Department.

Good morning, Chairman Jeffords and other members of the committee. We at the Department of Education are pleased that you have called this hearing to discuss the future of assistive technology and universal design. Assistive technology is critical in the lives of those of us with disabilities. The great scientist, Steven Hawking, personifies the potential that continues to be fulfilled through the use of assistive technology. Dr. Hawking uses an augmentative communication device. We can all take pride in that technology. The research in the use of a voice chip like the one in Dr. Hawking's device is part of what we support in the Department of Education through the National Institute on Disability and Rehabilitation Research.

There is a young man named Will McCarthy whom you all may remember. Will, who uses a sound board known as "The Liberator," joined us at the White House signing of the Individuals with Disabilities Education Act last June 4th. Because of this technological device, Will not only talked with the President but sang the President his favorite country and Western song.

I too know intimately the benefits of assistive technology. Activities of daily life that many of you take for granted, such as moving from this hearing room to your Chambers at the Capitol, may be impossible for someone like me who has no use of my legs. However, with assistive technology such as my wheelchair, with its motor and a driving stick, I am able to make that journey without too much difficulty. In fact, I can probably get there as fast or faster than most people in this room.

With the right assistive technology, the world of disabled individuals is incredibly broadening. The employment prospects and personal independence of disabled individuals can be significantly improved.

One thing is absolutely certain. Given the right tools, disabled individuals can learn and work in equal measure alongside their non-disabled peers. Assistive technology and universal design are the right tools.

NIDRR, although small in staff and budget compared to the National Science Foundation or the National Institutes of Health, is the lead Federal agency in disability and rehabilitation research. NIDRR is recognized and called upon for expertise in assistive technology and universal design not only in the United States but throughout the world. It leads in facilitating innovation on the part of its grantees and researchers in the arena of technology-related research and development and assistive technology service and device delivery.

At the Department of Education, we are proud that the scope of NIDRR's programs spans all disabilities and all age groups. There are products focusing on very young children as well as senior citizens. There are projects on traumatic brain injury and burn management and aging that address the technology needs of individuals with motor, sensory and cognitive disabilities.

NIDRR-sponsored programs also span the complete spectrum of the research and development continuum. Soon, we will have the most visible example of NIDRR-funded research—the accessibility features included in Windows 98. In the beta version manual, Microsoft acknowledges the NIDRR-funded research at the University of Wisconsin as the driving force in bringing this about.

We know that technology must move beyond the research and development stage into the commercialization phase. The development of the augmentative communication technology used by Dr. Hawking and countless others was begun in part by a NIDRR-sponsored research facility. Research aimed at full commercialization of a product, supported through small business initiatives, has generated the establishment of a number of small businesses. Isn't this the type of forward thinking that makes this country the land of opportunity? Shouldn't that opportunity be available to all of us?

NIDRR plays a crucial role in coordinating Federal Government activities and extramural research activities by acting as a technology hub for stakeholders in the assistive technology and engineering fields. NIDRR promotes coordination of these activities across the entire Federal Government through the Interagency Committee on Disability Research. Created 25 years ago, the ICDR now has three subcommittees—disability statistics, medical rehabilitation and, most relevant to today's hearing, technology. The technology subcommittee has recently produced one of the most comprehensive and up-to-date compendia of rehabilitation-related technology research and development in the Federal Government.

I have been focusing on NIDRR's contribution to research, development commercialization and coordination. There are many other examples of NIDRR-funded research that ultimately provide real and direct benefits for individual with disabilities. But you and I know that these research and related activities are the forerunners of something that has an even more direct impact on the lives of disabled people. We need assistive technology support to live and work independently.

Some of the technological support is for individual use, and some is integrated into mainstream products, transportation, information systems and the built environment.

But even once technology appears in the marketplace, NIDRR's involvement continues. It administers a $36.1 million effort in assistive technology grants authorized by the Tech Act. NIDRR's projects work collaborative with Sate agencies to improve the provision, access and purchase of assistive technology for persons with disabilities of all ages. There are assistive technology programs in all 50 States, as well as the District of Columbia, Puerto Rico, American Samoa, Guam, and the Commonwealth of the Northern Mariana Islands, and the U.S. Virgin Islands.

Through activities that promote systems change, the 56 projects have come a long way from the early days. Back then, there was no structure or organization, and access to technology for people with disabilities was fragmented and limited.

The Tech Act has been the catalyst for some dramatic changes in thousands and thousands of people's lives. Individuals report more timely and appropriate access to assistive technology services and devices, as well as more information, advocacy and training than a decade ago. And we have had significant opportunities to demonstrate and try out new technologies.

If I may, Mr. Chairman, I want to highlight just a few of our Tech Act-related activities.

All 56 Tech Act projects have been instrumental in passing or revising at least one piece of consumer-responsive legislation at the State level which would improve access to assistive technology, such as lemon laws and changes to Medicaid purchasing regulations.

All Tech Act projects engage in statewide training of consumers and providers. In 1996 alone, close to 200,000 people were trained by the 56 projects.

Forty-seven of the projects have created equipment loan centers. This has dramatically improved our ability to borrow and try out equipment.

Thirty-six of the 56 Tech Act projects, or 64 percent, have created financial loan programs with private banking institutions for revolving or low-interest loans that increase access to assistive devices.

Later this spring, we expect to send to Congress an administration proposal that builds upon past Tech Act accomplishments. Although we are still developing our proposal, I can tell you that at a minimum, we will seek to extend the authority of the Tech Act so that all States may receive a full 10 years of funding. Under the current period of authorization, while some States will have received 10 years of funding, others will not.

We at the Department have conducted five public hearings to gather information and comments on the future needs for assistive technology devices and services. We also examined the systemic barriers to meeting those needs and information about successful approaches that have been used to remove barriers. We did this so that individuals who need assistive devices and services may be able to get them, particularly individuals with disabilities.

Access is essential for success and independence.

What we consistently heard at these hearings is that barriers and gaps continue to challenge those of us with disabilities. The technology and information explosion may be leaving disabled people behind. The technology infrastructure that we are shaping must build accessibility features up front, so that we do not lose flexibility down the road.

New software applications replace currently-marketed applications at a pace that exceeds current research capability to keep up with them. Blind people, for example, are having difficultly using the internet due to this situation.

Small business has minimal capital to feed back into research, and we need to find ways to stimulate markets.

Financing continues to be a major problem and may become more difficult in a managed care environment.

Expertise about technology and universal design is one of the Nation's most needed skills. It is critical for consumers of all ages, teachers, rehabilitation counselors, employers and services providers, to provide reasonable accommodations, evaluation and assessment services, maintenance, repair and upgrade. People want and need technology infrastructure that routinely provides information, training, awareness, demonstration and delivery, as well as research.

There is a continuing need for protection and advocacy services, particularly legal advocacy, on an individualized and systemic basis. This is especially true in a time of changes in third-party payments.

Many seniors and providers to seniors reminded us of the aging four population, with one American turning 50 every 7.6 seconds—I achieved this in December. We know from our research that as we age, we depend more and more on technology to assist us with chores of everyday living and learning, but we need more innovative technology to meet these needs.

Access to information about assistive technology and financing continues to be a significant problem, particularly in rural, hard-to-reach and minority communities.

Mr. Chairman, as these hearings proceed and as we contemplate reauthorization of the Tech Act, we all must keep a few questions in mind. First, how has the world of technology changed in the past decade?

Two, what do we need to do in order to provide access to assistive technology in the 21st century for individuals with disabilities?

Three, how do we assure universal design of all technology, especially information and telecommunications?

Four, what tools do we need to sustain technology across the life span, individually and collectively?

Five, what expertise will be required to meet the challenge of rapid technological change and more modest but necessary challenges for maintenance, repair and upgrade of technology?

And six, how will we finance assistive technology, not only today, but in the future?

Our continuing role in assistive technology in the 21st century is clear. We must support crucial systemic change and the removal of barriers. But we also must provide the framework to meet challenges and to be leaders in the Information Age.

Mr. Chairman and members of the committee, we want to thank you all for the work that you have done. We are really excited, also, about the tech fair that you are going to be having this afternoon. And we look forward to any questions that you may have.

[The prepared statement of Ms. Heumann follows:]

PREPARED STATEMENT OF JUDITH E. HEUMANN

INTRODUCTION

Good morning, Chairman Jeffords, members of the committee. We, at the Department of Education, are pleased that you have called this hearing to address the needs for assistive technology and universal design into the 21st century.

Assistive technology is critical in the lives of those of us with disabilities. The great scientist, Steven Hawking, personifies the potential that continues to be realized through the use of assistive technology. Dr. Hawking uses an augmentative communication device to communicate his science to us. Americans can take special pride in that technology. The research in the use of a voice chip like the one in Dr. Hawking's device is part of what we support at the Department of Education through the National Institute on Disability and Rehabilitation Research (NIDRR).

And there's a young man named Will McCarthy. Will McCarthy, who uses a sound board known as the "Liberator," joined us at the White House signing of the Individuals with Disabilities Education Act (IDEA) last year. Without this technology, this young man would have no means of communicating with the world. Because of this technological device, Will not only talked with the President, but sang the President his favorite Country and Western song.

I, too, know intimately the benefits of assistive technology. Activities of daily life that many of you take for granted, such as moving from this hearing room to your chambers in the Capitol, may be impossible for someone like me who has no use of my legs. However, with assistive technology, such as my wheelchair with a motor and a driving stick, I am able to make that journey without too much difficulty. In fact, I can probably get there at a faster pace than you.

Today, I will talk about the technological changes and its impact on the need for assistive technology. I will share some of NIDRR's accomplishments and the Institutes' work with the Technology-Related Assistance for Individuals with Disabilities Act (Tech Act) and technology research. Guided by the challenge of change as expressed by those who testified at our five public Tech Act hearings—disabled people, business people, providers and State and local government staff—I will share with you what they have said about the needs of disabled people in the future. People who want to learn, work and contribute to community life. People who know that technology can, without a doubt, level the playing field. I know that is an important principle for you, Mr. Chairman, and the work of this Committee.

Through NIDRR, the Department of Education plays a leadership role in the nation's efforts in research and delivery of assistive technology and universal design.

NIDRR, although very small in staff and budget compared to the National Science Foundation or the National Institutes of Health, is the lead Federal agency in disability and rehabilitation research. NIRR is recognized and called upon for expertise in assistive technology and universal design not only in the United States but throughout the world. It leads in facilitating innovation on the part of its grantees and researchers in the arena of technology-related research and development and assistive technology service and device delivery.

The scope of NIDRR's programs encompasses all disabilities and all age groups. There are projects focusing on very young children as well as senior citizens. There are projects on traumatic brain injury and burn management and aging that address the technology needs of individuals with motor, sensory and cognitive disabilities. NIDRR manages a vast range of disability research associated with technology for all people with disabilities.

NIDRR-sponsored programs span the complete spectrum of the research and development continuum. The soon-to-be most visible example of NIDRR-funded research that really will make a difference in the lives of people with disabilities is the accessibility features included in Windows 98. In the beta version manual, Microsoft acknowledges the NIDRR-funded research at the University of Wisconsin as the driving force in bringing this about. Windows 98 is an example of NIDRR's leadership in universal design—the design of consumer products, transportation and information systems and the built environment that incorporates features so that people with all kinds of needs can use them.

The ramp, for example, is used by bicyclists, by parents pushing strollers and by wheelchair users. Captions on televisions are used by people in noisy settings, people for whom English is a second language and people who are deaf or have a learning disability. Voice activated phones can be used by people who are driving as well as visually impaired individuals.

NIDRR knows that technology must move beyond the research and development stage to commercialization. The development of the voice chip technology, that is used by Dr. Hawking and countless others, was begun, in part, by a NIDRR-sponsored research facility. Research aimed at full commercialization of a product supported through small business initiatives has generated the establishment of a number of small businesses. This is what makes this country unique and great.

NIDRR plays a crucial role in coordinating Federal Government activities and extramural research activities by acting as a technology hub, if you will, for stakeholders in the assistive technology and engineering fields. NIDRR promotes coordination of these activities across the entire Federal Government through the Interagency Committee on Disability Research (ICDR) which was created by statute in 1973. Recent years have seen an increase in the ICDR activities, and it now has three subcommittees: disability statistics, medical rehabilitation, and most relevant to today's hearing, technology. The technology subcommittee has recently produced one of the most comprehensive and up-to-date compendia of rehabilitation-related technology research and development in the Federal Government.

This first part of my testimony about NIDRR's contributions has focused on research, development, commercialization and coordination. There are many other examples of NIDRR-funded research that ultimately have real and direct benefit to individuals with disabilities. But you and I know that these research and related activities are the forerunner of something that has an even more direct impact on the lives of disabled people. Disabled people need technological support to live independently. Some of the technological support is for individual use and some of the technological support is integrated into mainstream products, transportation, information systems and the built environment.

Once technology appears in the marketplace, NIDRR's involvement continues with the administration of a $36.1 million effort in assistive technology grants authorized by the Tech Act. NIDRR's 56 projects work collaboratively with state agencies to improve the provision, access, and purchase of assistive technology for persons with disabilities of all ages. There are assistive technology programs in all 50 States, the District of Columbia, Puerto Rico, American Samoa, Guam, the Commonwealth of the Northern Mariana Islands, and the U.S. Virgin Islands.

Through activities that promote systems change and improve the way we do the business of assistive technology service delivery, the 56 projects have come a long way from the early days. Back then there was no structure or organization, and access to technology for people with disabilities was fragmented and limited.

Agencies in each State that are responsible for the provision and training of assistive technology are working together so that every individual who might benefit from assistive technology is aware, kowledgeable, and has access to it.

The Tech Act has been the catalyst for some dramatic changes in thousands and thousands of individual lives. Individuals report more timely and appropriate access to assistive technology services and devices as well as more information, advocacy and training than a decade ago. And, we have had significant opportunities to demonstrate and try out new technologies.

If I may, Mr. Chairman, I want to highlight just a few of our Tech Act related successes:

- All 56 Tech Act projects have been instrumental in passing or revising at least one piece of consumer-responsive legislation at the State level which would improve access to assistive technology, such as lemon laws and changes to Medicaid purchasing regulations.
- All Tech Act projects engage in statewide training of consumers and providers. In 1996, close to 200,000 persons were trained by the 56 projects.
- 47 of 56 projects have created equipment loan centers. This has dramatically improved our ability to borrow and try out equipment.

• 36 of 56 Tech Act projects, or 64 percent, have created financial loan programs with private banking institutions for revolving or low-interest loans that increase access to assistive devices.

Later this spring, we expect to send to the Congress an Administration proposal that builds upon past Tech Act accomplishments. Although we are still developing our proposal, I can tell you that, at a minimum, we will seek to extend the authority of the Tech Act so that all States may receive a full 10 years of funding as was contemplated in fiscal year 1994. Under the current period of authorization, some States will have received 10 years of funding, while others will not.

We at the Department have conducted five public hearings to gather information and comments on the future needs for assistive technology devices and services, the systemic barriers to meeting those needs, and information about successful approaches that have been used to remove barriers so that individuals who need assistive devices and services may be able to get them, particularly individuals with disabilities.

What we consistently heard is that barriers and gaps continue to challenge those of us with disabilities:

• The technology and information explosion may be leaving disabled people behind. The technological infrastructure that we are building must have accessibility features included at the outset. New software applications replace currently marketed applications at a pace that exceeds current research capability to keep up with them. Blind people, for example, are having difficulty using the Internet.

• Small business has minimal capital to feed back into research.

• Financing continues to be a major problem.

• Expertise about technology and universal design is one of the Nation's most needed skills, for consumers of all ages, teachers, rehabilitation counselors, employers and service providers in order to provide reasonable accommodations, evaluation and assessment services, maintenance, repair and upgrade. People want and need a technology infrastructure that routinely provides information, training, awareness, demonstration and delivery as well as research.

• Industry and consumers need a place to come together in order to demonstrate and market technology.

• There is a desperate need within the provider community for more skilled professionals to modify cars and vans.

• There is a continuing need for Protection & Advocacy services, particularly legal advocacy of an individualized and systemic nature, especially in a time of changes in third party payments.

• Many seniors and senior providers reminded us of the aging of our population, as one American turns 50 every 7.6 seconds. We know from our research that as we age we depend more and more on technology to assist us with chores of everyday living and learning; but we need more innovative technology to meet the needs.

• Access to information about assistive technology and financing continues to be a significant problem particularly in rural, hard-to-reach and minority communities.

Mr. Chairman, as these hearings proceed, and as we contemplate reauthorization of the Tech Act, we all must keep a few key questions in mind:

1. How has the world of technology changed in the past decade?

2. What do we need to do in order to provide access to assistive technology in the 21st Century for individuals with disabilities?

3. How do we assure universal design of ALL technology—especially information and telecommunications?

4. What tools do we need to sustain technology across the life span, individually and collectively?

5. What expertise will be required to meet the challenge of rapid technological change and the more modest but necessary challenges of maintenance, repair and upgrade of technology?

6. And, how will we finance assistive technology into the future?

A vision of our continuing role in assistive technology in the 21st century must support crucial systemic change and the removal of barriers. But, it also has to provide the framework to meet and lead in the Information Age.

Conclusion

Mr. Chairman & Members of the Committee, as I close, I again remind you of Stephen Hawking, Will Mccarthy and countless others throughout the United States. We use assistive technology and universal design to change the world for the better and simply to live in it, to work it and to learn.

The U.S. Government has a long and distinguished tradition of establishing and funding programs to aid Americans with disabilities. In the past several decades, these programs have evolved into critical tools designed to facilitate the independence and self-sufficiency of people with disabilities so we may have full access to and live productively within the mainstream of our communities.

You now have the opportunity to continue that commitment. I look forward to working with you on realizing a vision for the 21st century of technology that works for all Americans.

The CHAIRMAN. Thank you very much.

I want to acknowledge the presence of Senator Frist and also Senator Hutchinson, who has been very, very helpful in this area.

And now, I will turn to Senator Harkin for his opening statement.

OPENING STATEMENT OF SENATOR HARKIN

Senator HARKIN. Mr. Chairman, thank you very much. I apologize for being a few minutes late, but I heard most of Secretary Heumann's testimony. I want to thank all of you for being here today.

I was proud to be the chief Senate sponsor of the Tech Act in 1988. I worked with the chief sponsor on the House side, whose name was Congressman Jeffords; so it is nice to be in the same forum with you as we revisit this issue this year, Mr. Chairman. So thank you again for your longtime interest and support of assistive technology. It has been just wonderful to work with you through the years.

I want to thank Secretary Heumann and her staff for what they have done to implement the vision that we had back in the 1980s on assistive technology, and especially the staff of the Tech Act Projects, as well as advocates and consumers around the country. I am looking forward to the new legislation and to seeing what we can do to expand our efforts.

Again, this is an issue that has concerned me for a long time. Back in the 1970s, I was on the House Science and Technology Committee, when we first started doing some initial grants and investments in assistive technology. At that time, Mr. Chairman, I joined Senator Jennings Randolph—I think it was 1977 or 1978—in delivering to then President Carter the first closed caption decoder at the White House. We have come a long way since then, but my interest in this goes back a long way. I have seen the differences it has made in the life of my own brother—the assistive technology that enables him to live by himself and have a full life and to be able to socialize. Not only that, but before he retired from his job, had it not been for some of the assistive technology devices that he used, I do not think he could have remained independent.

My nephew, who was injured in the Navy, is quadriplegic. I see how he gets around with a lift on his van, driving around as he does, being able to work, and using all the devices he has around his house.

I am reminded also of a farmer in Iowa, Don Wolford. Don is a paraplegic, and he farms 1,100 acres. He has a lift that literally lifts him onto his tractor, and he has hand controls with which he can drive his tractor, and he farms 1,100 acres. Without assistive technology, he would not be able to do it.

Then, there is my young friend, Danny Piper, who has Down's syndrome. He works a full-time job, but he has diabetes, so he has a special watch that beeps to remind him when he has to have a snack to keep his blood sugar level intact.

So it is not just Steven Hawking, although we are very proud of him, but there are lots of people out there whose daily lives have been made better because of the technology that is now available.

The assistive technology research that NIDRR is doing really has many spillover effects. We always hear about how defense research spills over into the private sector, and the same is true here. I saw a television commercial the other day advertising voice-activated software for business executives. That technology was originally developed for people whose disability kept them from using a keyboard, for example.

I was also the author of the bill that mandated that all of the television sets in the United States with a size 13-inch screen or bigger have a chip in them—and I remember the fight on that one. Obviously, I have thought of it in terms of my own brother and the deaf community in the United States, that they could not take this big box with them, and we had information from the chip manufacturers that they could make this little chip for practically nothing. I will not bore you with all the details, but having done that, we find now that it is not just the deaf community that uses it—it is hard-of-hearing people, it is business people—the sports bars love these things—English as a second language, which you mentioned, Ms. Heumann. I saw a demonstration where they were using "Sesame Street" in Spanish and then putting the English subtitles down below, so that kids could listen and follow in the English language.

So the spillover of this has been just great, and it is not just the disability community. So I hope that in discussing the funding for assistive technology, and especially for NIDRR, we will keep in mind that it has much broader application. It may start with the disability community, but it has much broader application than just that.

So there have been a lot of changes in technology since we started out, Jim, back in the eighties, and whatever we can do to take the bill now, as it sunsets, and get a new bill out there and push the horizons of this research, is what we have got to do, and I appreciate your leadership on it and thank you very much.

The CHAIRMAN. Well, thank you for your comments. It has been tremendous working with you over the years.

Senator Frist, do you have some comments?

OPENING STATEMENT OF SENATOR FRIST

Senator FRIST. Thank you, Mr. Chairman. I will be very, very brief and simply thank you for holding the hearing today and for taking the lead on legislation to replace the Tech Act, which will sunset at the end of this year.

As chairman of the Subcommittee in the Commerce Committee on Science, Technology, and Space, I have a particular interest in technology and communication and how technological tools can be used to facilitate communication and interaction among individuals.

Assistive technology has clearly had a huge impact and with advances in technology will make an even greater impact in the future.

I particularly today want to thank Chairman Jeffords for inviting my good friend Carol Smith from Knoxville, TN, who will be testifying a little later today.

Thank you for holding this hearing, Mr. Chairman.

The CHAIRMAN. Thank you, Senator Frist.

Senator Wellstone.

OPENING STATEMENT OF SENATOR WELLSTONE

Senator WELLSTONE. Thank you, Mr. Chairman.

I had a really brilliant statement, but Senator Harkin started talking to me, and I have forgotten every word.

The CHAIRMAN. I do not believe that for a minute. [Laughter.]

Senator WELLSTONE. The part about "brilliant" is what you do not believe. [Laugher.]

I actually in 30 seconds want to say two or three things. First of all, to Secretary Heumann, my apologies. I was desperately trying to finish up at meeting, and I apologize for missing your testimony. I think we are very lucky to have your leadership. You are so skillful, and I thank you.

The second thing I want to say is that this is a huge issue to Minnesota. As Senator Harkin knows, Governor Perpich, who is no longer with us, started talking about assistive technology, and I think part of what was done in Minnesota was the precursor of some of the really good national work. The STAR Program is very important in our State, and I have been to so many moving meetings. I remember a woman who was a very successful businesswoman saying, "The only difference between my being able to get out of bed, get dressed, go to work, be a successful entrepreneur and contribute to the community and live a life with dignity and not being able to do all of those things is this assistive technology, and the thing that I worry about is whether or not it will be available for all the people who can use it to be able to have full lives." And I think that is what this is about.

Then, my final point, which is why I asked you for this privilege, is that I just want to say that one of the reasons I really love this guy is because of his commitment. We have a terrific chair—I am very sorry he is a Republication—but with the exception of that, and that is a big exception, he is a wonderful chair. But the reason why I really love this guy is because of his absolute passion and advocacy and leadership and courage, not so much for the developmental disabilities community, but with the community.

The CHAIRMAN. Thank you very much.

Now, let me turn to you to get some more information on your activities and what you are doing. In addition to publishing the Compendia on Rehabilitation Technology, does the Inter-Agency Committee on Disability Research have the power to promote increased coordination in federally-funded research on assistive technology and increased consistency in Federal policies with regard to funding and services related to assistive technology? How does this work, and what do you do in that area?

Ms. HEUMANN. I would like Kate Seelman to start answering the question and give you some information about the Interagency Coordinating Council on Disability, because she chairs that, and then we will go from there.

The CHAIRMAN. Fine. That is acceptable.

Ms. SEELMAN. Good morning, Senator.

The Interagency Committee on Disability Research promotes collaboration and promotes information exchange and coordination. The Interagency Committee on Disability Research has three subcommittees—one on disability statistics, one on medical rehabilitation, and one on technology.

The technology subcommittee is co-chaired by the National Science Foundation and NIDRR and incorporates membership within it of the major Federal agencies that contribute to rehabilitation research, including the Department of Veterans Affairs, the Federal Laboratory Consortium, NASA, and other like agencies—the National Center for Medical Rehabilitation Research in the medical and bioengineering area. The subcommittees meet every second month, and mainly, since they are young, they have been doing work in information exchange and in compendium-building, to understand exactly what the Federal Government is supporting at this particular point.

The CHAIRMAN. Do you think we need to alter the legislation in any way to improve, or does there need to be improvement in the exchange of information, in the States as well as the Federal agencies?

Ms. HEUMANN. I think it is certainly something that we would be more than glad to talk with your staff about. Certainly, I think that coordination around research is appropriate. I think we have been working on doing more effective coordination at the policy level and around funding issues and exchange information, and I think the way the ICDR is currently structured, we currently would not have as broader an authority as you are discussing right now.

The CHAIRMAN. In your testimony, you support 10 years of Federal funding for each State Tech Project. All 50 State Tech Projects have developed identities and are seen as a resource in their respective States. If we were to authorize Federal funding for limited core activities for Tech Projects that have exceeded 10 years of Federal funding, which core activities are the most important?

Ms. HEUMANN. I think we believe that information exchange is certainly critically important. Being able to continue to look at financing issues is very important. The issue of technology and information exchange, and the ability also to be able to continue to stay on top of the changing fields and to continue to have influence over how fields making themselves accessible, I think is also critically important.

The area of professional development is another issue that we believe is very important, because we believe that there are insufficient numbers of people who are trained to be able to actually assist disabled individuals in obtaining the kind of technology that they need.

Those would be some of the issues that we think would need to continue to be emphasized.

The CHAIRMAN. We look forward to working with you on those.

Medicaid, managed care organizations and school districts have different terminology for some assistive technology devices and services. The result is that if an inappropriate term is used in one context, a person may be denied funding for needed assistive technology. This does not appear to be a good idea. How do we correct that?

Ms. HEUMANN. During 1996 and 1997, NIDRR developed National Classification System of assistive technology devices and services as required by Title II of the Tech Act legislation. The classification system was developed in consultation with other Federal agencies, State agencies, and Tech Act projects, as well as other groups and individuals.

Also authorized under this legislation is a data collection activity, testing the classification system, that will collect nationally representative information about the availability, use, cost, and reliability of assistive technology. At this time, NIDRR is collecting information from professionals who provide assistive technology devices and services and consumers and family members who receive assistive technology devices and services. The information will be analyzed to examine the types of assistive technology and services provided to consumers, how those devices and services are funded, and how satisfied the consumers are with devices and services.

The CHAIRMAN. You mentioned in your statement that there might be a problem created by managed care having available devices or whatever else. Could you expound on that?

Ms. HEUMANN. Yes. There are a number of things that we have been hearing for many years, but I think the issue became more apparent as Dr. Seelman was conducting the five hearings that I mentioned in my testimony over the last few months.

We have been hearing that managed care providers are not necessarily enabling disabled individuals to get the technology that they need. There are cost restrictions. Individuals who are the providers do not necessarily understand the importance of the technology, the cost implications down the road if individuals do not get that technology.

And if I could give an example—and then I want to let Kate give you some more information on this—for someone like myself who needs an adapted seating system, I can be required to get something, or the managed care company could pay for various types of seating systems. But if they were to give me an off-the-shelf seating system, it could produce many different problems down the road. An individual with a spinal cord injury who, for example, sat on a $30 to $50 cushion, it would be a cheap cushion, but if that individual is prone to decubiti ulcers, it could result in $30,000 to $50,000 worth of costs in the future.

So some of the Tech Act programs have been working within their States, helping to provide greater information to the managed care providers in the State to get them to understand the importance of this issue, but we see it as a growing problem.

Ms. SEELMAN. The National Institute on Disability and Rehabilitation Research, showing the complementarity between the research program and the Tech Act, established a Managed Care Rehabilitation Research Training Center to address what our constituencies have seen across rehabilitation as a very serious problem.

The Tech Acts themselves, with Missouri and other States as leads, have been doing managed care studies and working with providers, which will have to go on into the future because it is such a dynamic marketplace.

People who gave witness—I remember in particular a pediatrician who said that managed care can be explained in two words—paper work. In any case, he expressed extraordinary problems with getting technology to children and extraordinary support for the Tech Act. Providers apparently do not know, as Judy Heumann said, and are not familiar with technology and the importance of technology for independence—the new providers in the managed care environment.

The CHAIRMAN. Senator Harkin.

Senator HARKIN. Thank you, Mr. Chairman.

Again, I would just join the others in thanking you, Judy, for your wonderful leadership in all areas down at OSERS, but especially in technology and in NIDRR. We just thank you so much, and hopefully, with this new legislation, we can really expand some of the things we have been doing.

There are a couple of things that always bothered me, or plagued us, I guess, in terms of how we get some of this assistive technology to rural areas. We have always had a problem in those small communities. I know there is not a simple answer, and there are many challenges, and I am just asking the broader question of have you been keeping on top of this, and do you have any suggestions or advice for us as to how we might look at how we can get more technology assistance to rural areas?

Let me also just say that when we did this bill back in 1988 and when we did it again in 1994, we talked about the costs of some of these things, and I remember talking about the inaccessibility in rural areas. At that time, we talked about setting up in States repositories of assistive technology devices and so on which people might be able to draw down and use at various times. I do not know if anything ever came of that. Is that being done at all, and was that successful or not?

Ms. HEUMANN. I think you would actually be very excited by some of the work that the States in fact are doing. Obviously, in some States, issues affecting the rural communities are more prevalent than others, so in a State like Iowa, rural issues certainly are looked at.

Let me just flash this for you. We have materials that are designed by one of our TA providers that gather information from across the Tech Act programs and basically highlight some of the successes. There is a nice little "cheat sheet" in the middle of this which outlines regional centers, equipment loan programs, equipment exchange and recycling programs, for example. Most of the Tech Act programs have regional centers now, regional centers meaning that they can have more than one office, they can provide funding to other organizations like independent living centers and other types of programs where those projects can be involved in providing individuals with information about funding-related issues, how to get technology, how to make the various funding sources work for you.

Also, many of the Tech Act programs—actually, most of them—have web sites. So that for individuals who have access to computers, web sites are very helpful because they can get greater information. In a State like Washington, their Tech Act program was specifically involved in helping to set up 22 libraries so they would be accessible for disabled individuals from across the States.

A number of the centers' programs that I have visited, for example, actually give people the opportunity to try technology, to borrow it, to take it home, which I think is very important. In the 1970s, when I first started doing some international travel, I was really impressed with some of the programs in Scandinavia, where they had many programs throughout their countries where individuals could go, without anyone trying to sell them any equipment, and try out different things. While we are not on that scale through the Tech Act programs, I think it is of proven value to let people try something, take it home, and if it does not work, they do not have to look at buying it, and if it does work, they can.

Senator HARKIN. It looks like you have one in almost every State, though.

Ms. HEUMANN. That is right. We have Tech Act programs now in every State and the Territories.

Kate wanted to comment.

Ms. SEELMAN. I did want to speak both to the rural area and stretch out a little bit from the rural area, because of the sparsity of population and great distances. I think that the public hearing spoke to a lot of problems, especially perhaps in the Midwest and in the South, and one of the many answers looking into the future, it seems to me, is the establishment from the research program of tele-rehabilitation engineering and application of telecommunication in the delivery of services remotely.

Since the States are now all gearing up in terms of telecommunications infrastructure in health and education and commerce, it will be very important in the future to assure the accessibility of that infrastructure for our older population, for people with disabilities and for others.

Another issue that acme out very clearly in the hearings, especially in the rural areas, was the struggle with small business. There, the size of the markets comes out very clearly.

These are two areas, and again, the telecommunications and building a telecommunications infrastructure also goes right to the wonderful concept of universal design, which we are all hearing much more about. If you can design this infrastructure for all people, then we will save money.

Ms. HEUMANN. In our office, for example, a couple of weeks ago, we could not get an interpreter to be able to on site for a meeting, but we were able through telecommunications to have interpreters off-site, in our office, being able to scan the room and see who was speaking using the interpreters. It is really wonderful.

Ms. SEELMAN. Let me just say one more thing, because I think Senator Frist would be interested in this. We have a demonstration in relation to our spinal cord injury centers where visiting nurses are taking telecommunications equipment into remote areas so that they are imaging the decubitus ulcer, sending it back to the area where all the physicians and experts are focused. They look at it, they measure it, and they send back their recommendation of how to treat it in a very rural area.

The same thing can happen with evaluations and assessments in rural areas for kids and adults with disabilities.

The CHAIRMAN. Thank you. The lights are not working, so I am going to have to pass you a little slip of paper. I would remind you that we have four panels to hear from today.

Senator Frist.

Senator FRIST. Thank you, Mr. Chairman.

I will limit my questioning to one question to Secretary Heumann or Dr. Seelman, either one. In your statement, you referred to "universal design." Could you elaborate for the committee on what universal design encompasses, what it means, and why it is so important?

Ms. SEELMAN. Universal design is essentially designing consumer products, transportation, communication and the built environment for the broadest range of function. That is essentially what it means. Universally-designed—it is a democratic idea that all of our products and our systems will be accessible.

It is cheaper to do it at the design stage than to come back and retrofit as we have had to do with television systems. I am very hard of hearing, and we had to retrofit the television system with captioning, and it was an old technology that we had to superimpose captioning on. One would hope that if you could design early on—and of course, one of the early example of universal design is the one that Senator Harkin mentioned—the decoder, where you put the chip in the television, and it is a mainstream technology. Everybody buys it; mother or whoever has a little hearing problem switches it on, uses vision and hearing, or one or the other. That is the genius of universal design.

We have two engineering centers that have addressed universal design for quite some time, one in Wisconsin, and in fact, the PI there was referred to as "the Moses of universal design." And then we have a built environment leader, Ron Mace, who has long been involved in universal design in the built environment.

We have a long way to go, but it is a powerful vision.

Ms. HEUMANN. Curb cuts and ramps are great examples. We had so many difficulties getting curb cuts in the beginning, and now, it is fascinating to just stand on a corner and watch who uses curb cuts—men and woman pushing baby carriages, kids using rollerskates, people with bicycles. If you go to Japan, they have curb cuts throughout the country having nothing to do with disabilities because so many people use bikes that they just automatically built them into their environment.

Senator FRIST. Thank you.

The CHAIRMAN. Thank you.

Senator Wellstone.

Senator WELLSTONE. Thank you, Mr. Chairman.

Madam Secretary, I think I am going to take three questions and, following Senator Frist's lead, try to make them one question.

I am interested in trying to zero in on what, over the last 20 or 30 years, these improvements have meant in personal terms in people's lives. Second, I am interested in how you would prioritize the two or three or four things that we have absolutely got to do as you think about the direction in which we are going with this piece of legislation. And third—and this may be the most troubling question—given the scope of the bill, are we really providing assistance in this Act to all those in this country who need it, and if we are not, why not?

In other words, we start with the positive and talk about the priorities and where we need to go, but then I have to ask the question—quite often, here in committee, and I do not fault anyone for this, we hear testimony, we are moved by it, I think we are all committed to this, and then we end up saying, given the reality, we have this amount by way of resources to spend. And I sometimes think, well, wait a minute—who defined that reality? That is why I ask you the last question—will we be serving all the people who need it, and if not, why not?

Ms. HEUMANN. Well, the Tech Act was never designed as a piece of legislation to ensure that all individuals in fact got services. The real intent of the Tech Act in part was to make sure that, first, people begin to understand about appropriate technology and how it could be applied for disabled people, reaching out into the disability community, allowing them to have a better understanding of the technology that in fact was out there, to help identify the unmet needs and who needed the services.

Senator WELLSTONE. And once people know, then——

Ms. HEUMANN. Well, then, there is the Tech Act itself, specifically. There are many different pieces of legislation that are supposed to help assure that people get the equipment, but in part, they are supposed to be networking with school districts and State departments of rehabilitation and working with State agencies like the State departments of help, helping them identify policies that may need to be corrected, or helping to make adjustments prior to legislation actually coming into effect.

They are doing things like helping lemon laws to be passed when they are identifying problem. I think you will see that States are doing different types of work, focusing on different populations, but the truth of the matter is that this legislation being passed will not result in all people getting services, but what this legislation has really been helping is greater numbers of disabled individuals and their families to become aware of what is out there. And I think it has also resulted in the designers of technology getting a better understanding of the fact that disabled people are a very vibrant part of the consumer community and how it is very important for them to be taking the needs of disabled people into consideration.

Senator WELLSTONE. Could I amend my question, then? This piece of legislation is vitally important for what it does. That is what you are saying.

Ms. HEUMANN. Yes.

Senator WELLSTONE. If it is not outside the scope of your testimony today, I guess what I am interested in is as we look to different States and what is being done and what is not being done, and we know how important assistive technology is to enriching people's lives, ennobling people's lives, and empowering people, are we anywhere close to where we should be, or not?

Ms. HEUMANN. Well, as someone who has passed the 50-year-old mark and had my disability when I was a year and a half, I think we have certainly gone much further, both in the design of technology—because when someone wanted to give my parents a motorized wheelchair for free when I was 12 years old, and they would not take it, it was one of the first times that someone even would have had a motorized wheelchair—but now you see young children with motorized wheelchairs, because the concept of a motorized wheelchair has changed. People recognize the fact that disabled children and adults who are not able to move their wheelchairs freely and independently are restricted by not being able to get a motorized wheelchair, which gives them greater access to move around.

So I think we have been elevating the discussion. I think that when we look at States like Missouri and Massachusetts which have been able, through their Tech Acts, to work on getting State legislation passed to assure that as State agencies are purchasing computers and software, it is accessible to all individuals, blind individuals, deaf individuals. That is a major problem.

Some of you may have seen the article in the paper today about "Y2K," the year 2000 issues. We are very concerned about the fact that lots of technology out there is not accessible and that as Sates and local communities and the Federal Government are moving into upgrading their equipment, that the equipment that they are going to be purchasing be accessible. And the Tech Acts are vehicles that are really trying to put pressure in their States to assure that designers are building into the basic framework. They are leveragers. I think that that is very important, to see these programs as leveragers.

Senator WELLSTONE. Thank you.

Thank you, Mr. Chairman.

The CHAIRMAN. Senator Murray—and you can finish your questioning by introducing the next panel.

Senator MURRAY. Thank you, Mr. Chairman. I really appreciate it.

Judy, thank you to you and your Department for the excellent job you do with the changing technology. I appreciate your mentioning the Washington State libraries, which have done an excellent job.

I recently met with the Lighthouse for the Blind, which is a consortium that, through assistive technology, has employed blind and deaf individuals with the Boeing Company. So there are some good things going on out there, and I just want to thank you for the job that you have done.

I know you have another panel coming up, Mr. Chairman, so I will save my comments for that panel, but thank you.

Ms. HEUMANN. Thank you.

The CHAIRMAN. Thank you both for your excellent help and very enlightening testimony. We will continue to work with you to try to improve as we go along.

Ms. HEUMANN. And thank you all for your great staffs; it is great to work with them.

The CHAIRMAN. Our next witness is Sam Jadallah, who will be more fully introduced by Senator Murray.

Senator MURRAY. Mr. Chairman, thank you for assembling this very impressive cross-section of witnesses today. I think this hearing is going to shed a very positive light on the remarkable role that technology plays in providing every individual every opportunity to contribute to our society, no matter what the job is.

Mr. Chairman, we have worked together to stress technology in almost every bill that this committee has reported out, and I was really pleased to help push this incredible resource with my colleagues, particularly technology for teacher training in the recent higher education reauthorization bill.

Networks like the Washington Assistive Technology Alliance in Seattle have been providing resources for years that have put people back in the work force and harnessed an array of talents and productivity.

As many of you know, I represent a somewhat small software company located in Washington State, and I am pleased that representatives of Microsoft Corporation have traveled the 3,000 miles across the different and different times zones to be here with us today to share their work in the area of assistive technology.

It is my pleasure to introduce to this committee Mr. Sam Jadallah, who serves as the vice president of Microsoft's Organization Customer Unit. Mr. Jadallah leads this worldwide business division which focuses on the sales and marketing of Microsoft's nonretail channel, small and medium-size companies, and training for information technology professionals.

Microsoft is committed to being an industry model of accessible products and design, and Mr. Jadallah will touch on the company's work in accessibility over the last 10 years.

I would also like to introduce Greg Lowney, Microsoft's director of accessibility, and David Bolnick, their accessibility program manager, who will provide you with a very informative demonstration.

Mr. Chairman, I think we are all really interested in what this group has to present to us. I think we will find it very exciting. And they are pleased to have this discussion without any Department of Justice discussions attached to it. [Laughter.]

Again, Mr. Chairman, thank you, and I apologize—I will not be able to stay for the entire hearing, because I am negotiating on the conference committee on the supplemental. But we are very pleased to have you here. Thank you.

The CHAIRMAN. Thank you.

Mr. Jadallah, please proceed. We are very glad to have you here.

STATEMENT OF SAM JADALLAH, VICE PRESIDENT, ORGANIZATION CUSTOMER UNIT, MICROSOFT CORPORATION, REDMOND, WA, ACCOMPANIED BY GREG LOWNEY, DIRECTOR OF ACCESSIBILITY, AND DAVID BOLNICK, ACCESSIBILITY MANAGER, MULTIMEDIA AND COMMUNICATIONS

Mr. JADALLAH. Good morning. We are very pleased to be here. Thank you very much, Chairman Jeffords, Senator Harkin, and Senator Murray for the kind introduction.

First, on behalf of Microsoft, I would like to thank the committee for its invitation to participate at this morning's hearing. We welcome the opportunity to present an overview of our accessibility efforts. After my initial comments, both David and Greg will present a brief demonstration and actually show you some of the accessibility efforts that we have in our technologies.

Often, when people think about assistive technology, the computer is not the very first thing that comes to mind; but in fact, the personal computer is one of the most promising assistive devices there is today.

I have heard many people say that for people without disabilities, computers are useful, but for people with disabilities, they are essential. That is true not only because of the increasing importance of the PC both in the workplace and at home, but also because the internet is bringing together individuals and providing access to information previously unimaginable. In many ways, the potential of the PC and the internet is unlimited, as it can be the ultimate equalizer.

The real value is a person's idea. The digital market is how they create and share those ideas with others. That idea could be poetry, a business plan, the next big software product, or a community support program.

The technical challenge is for us and the industry to ensure that everyone has access to participate in this world.

Microsoft aims to be a leader in this effort. We are committed to furthering the computer's role as assistive technology in two ways—first, by removing the barriers to computer use, by making our products accessible to all users. This is not just about making it easier but about allowing people to discover the power of a personal computer for the first time. And second, we work to make computers everyday partners in people's lives by making computer inexpensive, flexible, and even taken-for-granted devices.

In short, we aim to help personal computers empower individuals to improve their lives.

Microsoft has been involved in accessibility for nearly 10 years, since about the same time as the start of the Tech Act. While we have made good progress, the challenge is large, and our efforts have not always met our or others' expectations. But we are a company very focused on customer feedback, and we believe that we are headed on the right track.

Our earliest efforts involved a set of software add-ins called the Access Pack, which was developed in private-public cooperation. Starting with Microsoft Windows 95 and Windows NT Version 4, the features of the Access Pack were extended and integrated into the operating system. As a result, every personal computer with Windows 95 or Windows NT 4 includes features specifically designed for individuals who have difficulty typing or difficulty using a mouse, who are deaf or hard-of-hearing, or who have moderately-impaired vision.

Windows 98, which is about to be released, will contain additional accessibility features, and the next release of Windows NT will include even more.

The integration of these capabilities provides software developers with a standard way to support accessibility devices. This allows them to release their products to market more quickly than they have in the past.

These accessibility features and hundreds of the adaptive hardware and software products made by other companies make computers accessible to a wide range of people. They include people who are blind or who, like my 5-year-old son, are deaf, or others who can communicate by only clicking a single switch.

At Microsoft, we are working to improve in a very fundamental way the manner in which assistive technologies can be incorporated into the incessant stream of technological advances. The evolution of PC computer programs in particular is so rapid that this category of assistive technology has had difficulty maintaining support for the new products that their customers want to use. It has not been uncommon for accessibility-focused products to be 12 to 18 months behind, frustrating both the market and the customer.

We set out to tackle that problem when we released Microsoft Active Accessibility last year. Active Accessibility provides software features which software developers can utilize to make their programs more accessible. Although still in its infancy, Active Accessibility already helps companies make products more accessible without compromising their ability to innovate and allows manufacturers to create even more effective accessibility aids.

The internet is another fast-changing technology that poses a challenge to people with disabilities, as you have heard this morning. So Microsoft has built into Internet Explorer an extensive array of accessibility features. In addition, we are addressing the accessibility of the World Wide Web with a software development tool that enables web sites and software developers to easily add captions and audio descriptions to multimedia sent over the internet. Much in the same way that Senator Harkin mentioned captions on televisions, we would like to provide that same capability on the personal computer. Now, deaf users can capture the audio track of a multimedia presentation that they have previous missed.

Notwithstanding our significant progress, we recognize that we have also made missteps in the accessibility area. We released an upgrade to Internet Explorer last year that omitted some accessibility features in earlier versions. We corrected most of those problems about a month later; however, we have still not fully released full support for Active Accessibility within Internet Explorer. Rest assured, we see that as a backward step that Microsoft is working very hard to reverse.

In fact, it is in part to address these issues that Bill Gates reaffirmed our commitment at what we called "Accessibility Day," which was held on the Microsoft campus in February of this year. Its purpose was to raise awareness among Microsoft employees that accessibility must be a fundamental way we do software design. Bill also announced a five-point plan to guide our accessibility efforts in the future. A copy of this five-point plan, along with a statement of Microsoft's accessibility policy, has been submitted to the committee.

The five-point plan recognizes that Microsoft cannot go alone. Our efforts in the assistive technology area must be consolidated with those of the industry, disability organizations and advocates, and also the Government.

As part of the plan, we are taking additional internal steps this year to integrate individuals with disabilities into our product development process. We have already established and independent access review board to review the accessibility of our products, and we are also creating an advisory council to help ensure our product development efforts are on track.

In addition, we are strengthening promotion of accessibility in the marketplace by further enhancing the "Designed for Windows" logo program. The logo program sets out the minimum requirements that software developers must meet in order to brand their products as "Designed for Windows." We are attempting to raise the bar with respect to accessibility for both Microsoft and third party developers. We hope that our efforts with accessibility in software increase the employability of the disabled and lower the accommodation costs for employers everywhere.

Even with the progress that Microsoft and other companies have made in accessibility, there are significant challenges for everyone. First, there are a few hundred small companies and nonprofit organizations working on very creative and very targeted computer-based accessibility solutions. We must ensure that these idea incubators continue to have the support they need to keep up with the rapidly-changing technologies.

Second, there are tens of thousands of companies creating computer applications, equipment and content, and we must help them learn why it is important to make their products accessible and how to do so. In this respect, Microsoft feels that full adherence to section 508 of the Rehabilitation Act is an important step. Once commercial enterprises see that the major agency purchases are based on accessibility, as well as the rest of the feature set of a particular product, we will see great innovation in this area.

And third, there are millions of people with disabilities who can benefit from accessibilities of computer systems, but too many of them still do not have access to products that can make a significant difference in their lives. We must ensure that they, their trainers, their employers and educational institutions are fully informed of the range of solutions available.

Mr. Chairman, I have given you only a small glimpse of the accessibility efforts at Microsoft, and I also agree with Senator Harkin's comment that these aids provide broad support in addition to the disability community.

Disability advocates and Microsoft agree that there is still much to do, but we must not lose sight of the progress that we have made. We do not have to look far to see individuals once considered helpless who are now significant contributors to society. The remaining barriers will fall as industry, Government and the disability community continue to work together toward their common goals, and Microsoft is very committed to being an industry model and working to make our products accessible to the widest range of users. That is good business sense and good common sense.

Thank you.

[The prepared statement of Mr. Jadallah follows:]

PREPARED STATEMENT OF SAM JADALLAH, VICE PRESIDENT, ORGANIZATION CUSTOMER UNIT, MICROSOFT CORPORATION

Good morning, Mr. Chairman and members of the Committee. My name is Sam Jadallah. I am the Vice President of the Organization Customer Unit at Microsoft Corporation. I would also like to introduce two of my colleagues. Greg Lowney is Microsoft's Director of Accessibility. David Bolnick is an Accessibility Program Manager, who focuses on multimedia and communications applications.

On behalf of everyone at Microsoft, I want to thank the committee for its invitation to participate at this morning's hearing. We welcome this opportunity to provide you with an overview of our accessibility efforts. After my initial comments, Greg and David will give the Committee a brief demonstration of some of the assistive technologies that we have developed.

PC's are assistive technology

Often, when people think of assistive technology, the computer isn't necessarily the first thing that comes to mind. They think of wheelchairs, hearing aids, or guide dogs. But in fact the computer is one of the most promising assistive technologies there is today. That's true not only because of its increasing importance in both the workplace and home, but because so many people are striving to make computers easier to use and adaptable to individual needs.

Microsoft's commitment to being an industry model for accessible products

Microsoft is a leader in that effort. We are committed to furthering the computer's role as assistive technology in two ways. First, by removing barriers to computer use—by making our products accessible to all users. And second, by working toward the goal of computers as everyday partners in people's lives—by making computers inexpensive, diverse, even taken-for-granted devices that let all people work more efficiently, communicate more easily, and explore new worlds of information and entertainment.

As Microsoft's Chairman and CEO, Bill Gates, said before about 3000 Microsoft employees earlier this year, "our vision when we started the company was a computer on every desk and in every home." Mr. Gates went on to say that "the word to emphasize here is *every*."

Microsoft, thus, is committed to being an *industry model* for accessible products and design. We are committed to working with the numerous, specialized companies that build accessibility tools and technologies. And we are committed to being a leader among all software and computer companies in this area.

Microsoft's early efforts

Microsoft has been involved in accessibility for nearly 10 years. Our earliest efforts involved a set of software add-ins called the Access Pack, developed at the Trace R&D center at the University of Wisconsin-Madison with a grant from the National Institute on Disability and Rehabilitation Research.

Windows 95 and Windows NT 4.0

Starting with Microsoft Windows 95 and Windows NT 4 the features of the Access Pack were extended and built in. As a result, every PC with Windows 95 or Windows NT 4 includes features specifically designed for individuals who have difficulty typing or using a mouse, who are deaf or hard-of-hearing, or who have moderately impaired vision.

Windows 98, Windows NT 5.0, other MS products

Windows 98—which is coming soon—will contain additional accessibility features, and Windows NT 5.0 will include even more. Similarly, we have incorporated accessibility features into many of our other products, such as our word processor and our multimedia encyclopedia.

Keeping pace with the rapid evolution of PC's and their software

These accessibility features—and hundreds of adaptive hardware and software products made by other companies—make computers more accessible to a wide range of people. They include those who are blind or who, like Stephen Hawking, can communicate only by clicking a single switch.

At Microsoft, we are also working to improve—in a fundamental way—the manner in which assistive technologies can be incorporated into the incessant stream of technological advances. The evolution of PC computer programs, in particular, is so rapid that this category of assistive technology has had difficulty keeping up with the rest of the computer industry. We set out to solve that problem when we released Microsoft Active Accessibility 1.0 last year.

Active Accessibility 1.0

Active Accessibility provides software "hooks" which software developers can exploit to make their programs more accessible. Active Accessibility lets applications cooperate and communicate better with assistive technology, such as screen readers.

Although still in its infancy, Active Accessibility already helps companies make products more accessible without compromising their ability to innovate, and allows manufacturers to create more effective accessibility aids.

Internet and Internet Explorer 4.0, SAMI

The Internet is another fast-changing technology that poses a challenge to people with disabilities. So, Microsoft has built in to its Internet Explorer technologies an extensive array of accessibility features. In addition, Microsoft is addressing the accessibility of the World Wide Web with a software development tool called Synchronized Accessible Media Interchange—or "SAMI" for short—that enables webmasters and software developers to easily add captions and audio-descriptions to multimedia sent over the Internet.

A step back

Notwithstanding our significant progress, we recognize that we have made missteps in the accessibility area. We released an upgrade of our Internet Explorer technology last year that omitted the accessibility features in earlier versions. We corrected most of those problems about a month later, although unforeseen problems have further delayed full support for Active Accessibility within Internet Explorer. Rest assured, we see this as an unfortunate step backward that Microsoft is working to reverse.

Bill Gates reaffirms Microsoft's commitment to accessibility

In fact, it is in part to address these issues that Bill Gates reaffirmed our commitment at—what we called—"Accessibility Day," held on the Microsoft campus in February of this year. Its purpose was to raise awareness among Microsoft employees that accessibility must be a fundamental part of software design. Mr. Gates also announced a five-point plan to guide our accessibility efforts in the future. A copy of this five-point plan, along with a statement of Microsoft's accessibility policy has been submitted to the Committee along with the written version of my remarks.

The five-point plan recognizes that Microsoft cannot go it alone. Our efforts in the assistive technology area must be consolidated with those of the industry, disability organizations and advocates, and the government.

The scope of Microsoft's efforts

As part of the plan, however, we are taking additional, internal steps this year to integrate individuals with disabilities into our product development process. We have already established independent Access Review Boards to review the accessibility of our products from the viewpoint of specific disabilities. We also are creating an Advisory Council to help insure our product development efforts are on track with the needs of individuals with disabilities.

Logo guidelines

In addition, we are strengthening promotion of accessibility by further enhancing the "Designed for Windows" Logo program. The Logo program sets out minimum requirements that software developers must meet in order to brand their products as "Designed for Windows." Through the Logo program, we are attempting to raise the bar with respect to accessibility for both Microsoft and third-party developers.

Executive checklist

Internally, we are adding specific guidelines for the company in addressing accessibility in our products. When executives conduct product reviews, they will be able to use a checklist of features and best practices to address accessibility issues.

Increased resources

In addition, we are nearly tripling the number of Microsoft employees working full time on accessibility issues, to about 25 in all. Plus, many other employees at Microsoft are assigned to handle accessibility issues along with their other duties.

Our own HR efforts

I also want to say that, for Microsoft, accessibility is not just about the products we produce. It is also about empowering our own employees, so that they can achieve their fullest potential. At Microsoft, we are proud of the environment we have been able to create for employees with disabilities. We have a self-identification program that endeavors to meet the special needs of employees even before they join our company, and we have ongoing employee assistance and support programs.

A Challenge for All

Even with all the progress Microsoft and other companies have made in accessibility, there are significant challenges for everyone.

Idea "incubators" need continued support

• First, there are a few hundred **small companies and non-profit organizations working on very creative and very targeted computer-based accessibility solutions.** We must ensure that these idea incubators continue to have the support they need to keep up with rapidly changing technologies.

Innovation in assistive technology needs market place forces

• Second, there are tens of thousands of **companies creating computer applications, equipment, and content.** We must help them learn why it is important to make their products accessible, and how to do so. In this respect, Microsoft feels that full adherence to Section 508 of the Rehabilitation Act is an important step. Once commercial enterprises see that major agency purchases are based on accessibility, as well as on the rest of the feature set of a particular product, we will see great innovation in the area.

Assistive technology is only good if those in need have access to it

• Third, there are **millions of people with disabilities** who can benefit from accessibility of computer systems. But too many of them still do not have access to products that can make a significant difference in their lives. We must ensure that they, their trainers, employers, and educational institutions are fully informed of the range of solutions available.

In conclusion

Mr. Chairman, I have given you only a small glimpse of the accessibility efforts at Microsoft. Disability advocates and Microsoft agree that there is still much to do, but we must not lose sight of the progress we have made. You don't have to look far to see individuals, once considered helpless, who are significant contributors to society. The remaining barriers will fall as industry, government, and the disability community continue to work together towards our common goals.

Microsoft is committed to being an industry model and making our products accessible to the widest range of users. That's good business and common sense. Thank you.

SAM JADALLAH, VICE PRESIDENT, ORGANIZATION CUSTOMER UNIT, MICROSOFT CORPORATION

As vice president of Microsoft's Organization Customer Unit, Jadallah leads a worldwide business division focused on sales & marketing in three areas: Microsoft's non-retail channel, small and medium size companies, and Microsoft's training and outreach efforts for IT professionals.

Jadallah is responsible for forging strategic industry partnerships with the channel to reach mutual business customers. This includes guiding Microsoft's channel efforts such as the Microsoft Certified Solution Provider program and Microsoft Direct Access, which combined reach over 700,000 channel business in 49 countries and the Microsoft Certified Professional (MCP) program, the industry's leading credential carried by over 200,000 technical professionals worldwide. He is also responsible for sales and marketing to small and medium business segment, which represent over 40 percent of Microsoft's worldwide revenue base. Additionally, he leads the training and outreach efforts which skilled over 2 million IT professionals on Microsoft technology last year.

Prior to his current role, Jadallah held the role of general manager of worldwide business strategy for Steve Ballmer. For nearly 4 years prior, Jadallah was the general manager of corporate and developer support, where he lead the building of the award winning innovative customer support service for Microsoft's line of server products. Jadallah has held other sales, management, and technical positions since joining Microsoft in 1987.

Jadallah is involved with community activities and serves on the board of the Alexander Graham Bell Association of the Deaf, Washington Chapter.

Tel: 425 703-6558
Fax: 425 936-7329
E-mail: samjad@microsoft.com

GREG LOWNEY, DIRECTOR OF ACCESSIBILITY, MICROSOFT CORPORATION

Greg Lowney manages Microsoft's Accessibility and Disabilities Group, which he founded in 1992. The group coordinates efforts to make Microsoft products and services, and computers in general, more accessible to people with disabilities. Lowney is responsible for implementing Microsoft policy to meet the company's strategic goals:

Develop products, technologies and services that are accessible and usable by all people.

Build relationships with the disability community to help us better understand and respond to customer needs, and help them understand our what we are doing.

Equip and motivate the development community to produce great accessibility solutions.

Empower computer users with information to help them make informed choices about what to use, and make best use of products they have.

Lowney has managed a variety of projects, including drafting corporate policy on accessibility and guiding the development of accessibility components for the MS-DOS, Windows, and Windows NT operating systems. Lowney developed guidelines for accessible software and Web sites and was responsible for addressing accessibility in product documentation, customer service, support, and internal training. He was promoted to Director in February 1998.

Previously, Lowney was Senior Program Manager for the Microsoft Windows 3.1 and 3.0 operating systems. Lowney was responsible for core components such as the basic user interface, protected mode systems, and networking, as well as accessibility. Lowney joined Microsoft in December of 1986 as a test manager, after holding a variety of programming positions and serving as microcomputer support specialist for a large school district.

Tel: 425 936-8510
Fax: 425 936-7329
TTY: 425 936-2627
E-mail: greglo@microsoft.com
Web: http://microsoft.com/enable/

DAVID BOLNICK, ACCESSIBILITY PROGRAM MANAGER, MICROSOFT CORPORATION

David Bolnick is the Accessibility Program Manager for multimedia tools and applications, and telecommunications.

Key projects:

• SAMI (Synchronized Accessible Media Interchange) authoring format architecture for closed captioning and audio description of multimedia and Web presentations

• SAMI support in NetShow media player and SAMI Caption Authoring Tool

Microsoft representative:

• SMPTE (Society of Motion Picture and Television Engineers) committee for closed caption authoring

• TAAC (Telecommunications Access Advisory Council of the US Access Board) committee for drafting guidelines for Section 255 of the Telecommunications Act of 1996

• Advisory Council for HiP Magazine (for deaf and hard of hearing children and teenagers)

• Human Interface Technology Lab, University of Washington (research related to visual accessibility)

David Bolnick joined Microsoft in January of 1990. Before joining the Accessibility & Disabilities Group, he was a member of the User Interface Architecture and Windows Design teams responsible for the new look and feel of Windows. Prior to coming to Microsoft, Mr. Bolnick was a Research Fellow at the University of California, San Francisco. His main area of research was visual processing in the eye. He received his Ph.D. in Physiology in 1984 from the University of California, Davis. He loves books, loves to learn, and serves his community as a mohel. His wife is a Family Physician and they have three loving boys.

Tel: 425 936-8342
Fax: 425 936-7329
E-mail: davebo@microsoft.com
Web: http://microsoft.com/enable/

Microsoft's Accessibility Policy

The following policy was officially adopted by Microsoft Corporation in July of 1995, and announced by Paul Maritz at Microsoft's Accessibility Summit 95:

As a leader in the software industry, Microsoft Corporation recognizes its responsibility to develop products and information technologies that are accessible and usable by all people, including those with disabilities. We will devote the time and resources necessary to ensure that all users enjoy access to our products, technologies and services. It is the responsibility of everyone at Microsoft to deliver on this commitment.

To realize this vision, Microsoft will address the needs of people with disabilities during all phases of product planning, development and support. This includes:

• Establishing accessibility guidelines for use internally and by third-party developers.

• Working with the disability community to solicit and incorporate feedback when planning and developing products and services.

• Supporting developers of disability access technologies.

• Continuing to recruit qualified people with disabilities to contribute to product development efforts, services and corporate culture.

• Addressing known accessibility issues with products and services as they are updated.

Microsoft Accessibility Five-Point Plan

Microsoft's Strategy

Microsoft has a four-pronged approach to making computers more accessible, by:

• **Develop** products, technologies and services that are accessible and usable by all people. This includes normal usability issues such as supporting keyboard usage and different appearance schemes, and accessibility-specific features such as closed-captions and compatibility with accessibility aids.

• **Build relationships** with the disability community to help us better understand and respond to customer needs, and so they can understand what we're doing.

• **Equip and motivate** the development community to produce great accessibility solutions. We promote accessible design to application developers, and create new technologies that make it possible to create accessibility aids that are more robust, effective, and timely, and require less work.

• **Empower consumers** with information to let them make informed choices about what to use, and make best use of the products they have.

Five New Initiatives

We are announcing five new initiatives to help bring about these goals:

1. **Strengthening promotion of accessibility** through the Designed for Windows(r) logo program

• **Set minimum bar for both Microsoft and third-party** hardware and software

• **Already has requirements** and future requirements

• **Looking at several options** to strengthen this program

2. **Adding specific guidelines** for the company in addressing accessibility in its products

• **Product features** and **best practices**

• **Not required, but reinforced** by executive management through periodic review meetings.

3. **Increasing communication** between the disability-advocacy community and Microsoft product groups

• **Advisory Council** to help us prioritize our efforts appropriately and verify our progress

• **Product Review Boards** to advise on specific product features

• **Technical Product Manager** to work with accessibility vendors

• **Network of representatives** from product groups

• **Marketing efforts focus** on making sure people get the information they need

4. **Significantly increase resources** devoted to accessibility

• **More than doubling** the number of staff members working full-time on accessibility:

a) **Provide strong leadership** in the accessibility field, both within the company and throughout the industry.

b) **Continue developing core accessibility technologies** to improve their scope, timeliness, and quality.

c) **Proactively oversee the work being done by key groups within the company,** providing expertise on accessibility issues and serving as internal advocates within those product groups.

d) **Continue improving the company's relations** with the disability community, key advocacy groups, and adaptive hardware and software manufacturers.

• **Centralizing the group** to ensure continuity and focus while **members continue working in product groups** where they can be most effective

• **Establishing a Directorship** to be responsible for overall strategy and operations

5. **Achieving measurable improvements** in the accessibility of key Microsoft(r) products

• **New Windows accessories** for people with different types of disabilities

• **Office** keyboard support, high contrast visuals, and compatibility with accessibility aids

• **Internet Explorer** compatibility with accessibility aids using Active Accessibility(tm)

• **Visual Basic** compatibility with accessibility aids using Active Accessibility

The CHAIRMAN. Thank you for very excellent testimony, and we certainly commend you on the work that is being done.

Mr. JADALLAH. Before you start with questions, let us just give you a brief demonstration of some of the technology.

The CHAIRMAN. Yes. Please go ahead.

Mr. LOWNEY. Thank you very much.

Microsoft has built many features into our products that benefit people with a wide range of disabilities, and I only have time to show you a few glimpses of selected examples.

Let us take a person who is blind or has dyslexia and might have difficulty reading the screen. They would be running a screen-reader program that tells them the things that are going on on the computer screen. Microsoft has tried to make this process easier by creating active accessibility to the technology which Mr. Jadallah mentioned earlier.

So here, we have a little demonstration tool which is using active accessibility to figure out what it is that the computer is doing. In this case, Dave is selecting menu items from this menu, and every time one is selected, the tool is informed of this through Active Accessibility and came speak the name out loud for anyone who needs to hear it.

One of the sections in the Windows interface that we are navigating through right now is called Control Panel, and that is a place where you can adjust many different settings to customize the way the computer behaves. And here, you will see that there is actually one section called Accessibility Options within the Control Panel. That is where you can apply many things related to how a person types on the keyboard, how they use the mouse, how the screen is displayed in colors, or providing feedback for people who are deaf or hard-of-hearing.

Now, you might have trouble actually reading this text here because it is too small, so Microsoft has built into our next operating system, Windows 98, a product called the Screen Magnifier. This is a very low-end magnification product which allows a person to temporarily enlarge any text or graphics appearing on the screen. So that as you can see here, it makes it much larger and easier to read.

Now, a person who has severe low vision will probably want to buy a more comprehensive, full-featured commercial product to use in his or her own work station. But by building this into the basic operating system, we have made sure it exists as a fallback wherever the user goes, on any system.

Another place where we have built in accessibility rather than having it be an add-on is in our web browser, Microsoft Internet Explorer. Here is a typical web page from the Microsoft web site. It is designed to be very good for people with normal vision, but if you have trouble seeing it, you can actually take control of a presentation using the accessibility options that are built right into Internet Explorer.

In this case, we are going to go into the Accessibility section of the options and choose to make the text larger, the contrast higher, the text brighter, and also especially to highlight things like headings to make it easier for a person with learning disabilities to scan the page and get the idea of how the structure goes.

Not only for people with low vision, there are also features here for people with other types of disabilities. For example, if you cannot use a mouse, you can navigate this on any other web page using the keyboard. So that simply by hitting the tab key multiple time, you will see that he can navigate to each of the links, and they are in fact also highlighted to make it easier to see where you are working. And of course, if you do not like seeing it this way, with a touch of a button, you can go back to the original appearance and see the web page the way the author had originally intended.

The web is increasingly using not only text, but also other types of multimedia, and so Microsoft has created the SAMI technology, which allows anyone to enhance multimedia content with both closed captioning for people who are deaf or hard of hearing and also audio description for people who are blind.

What we are going to show you here is a kiosk demonstration that is being created by the U.S. Holocaust Memorial Museum here in Washington. This is actually an application that uses Internet Explorer and takes advantage of it to display the text and also to display videos and captions for those videos.

In this case, you can see that we are not only playing the video but displaying the captions just like you do on television. But because this is a computer, SAMI allows much more power than you have on your television, and the user can decide—if they do not like the way the captions are displayed, they can change them. They can make the font bigger, or they can even change the colors to have it displayed in a way which suits their visual needs.

In fact, SAMI can be used for many things beyond just captioning. So if we look at another section of this demonstration kiosk, there is a place where it will actually be showing text and reading this aloud, but at the same time it reads the text, it highlights the passage it is reading. What that does is allow a person who is just learning English or who has dyslexia or other reading disabilities to more easily follow along.

Those are just a few of the things that we have built into some our products. I hope this gives you an idea of the power of assistive technology to let people actually use, communicate, be productive in the workplace and in education.

Thank you very much.

The CHAIRMAN. Thank you. That was very, very helpful, and I commend you for it.

Let me turn to probably the greatest problem this Nation has right now in the sense of education, and that is illiteracy. I wonder what you can develop to increase the market to some 80 million people who are functionally illiterate and at the same time give us the tools to be able to provide remedial help to the schools or to individuals to learn how to read.

I know that IBM had a Writing to Read Program—I do not know what happened to it, but it has not blossomed into anything. What work do you do, or do you take these kinds of problems and try to study them?

Mr. JADALLAH. There are two areas that we are focusing in on, Senator. One is around generally working with academic institutions, K through 12 schools around the Nation, to readily help them utilize technology in the school systems, both in the public areas, such as libraries, but also in the school systems, where they can utilize technology to help teach and help students learn.

We have a number of innovative programs, including laptop programs, where we loan laptops or provide loans for laptops, where every student has one, and that is a way for them, even in the inner city, to have basically a learning tool.

Once there is a PC available in the school, there are a number of software efforts underway, both at Microsoft and with partners of Microsoft, to supply additional tools to help students learn. In fact, we use that quite a bit, and I am using it with my 5-year-old son today.

We also have another initiative that is focused around helping people utilize technology to enter into the technology field and recruiting people in other fields who are currently displaced or welfare-to-work and in other areas, who are really interested in getting into the technology field. And we have another imitative called Skills 2000, which is a very broad initiative focused around helping those people get into the workplace as well.

I cannot impress upon you how important that is to our society. The cost of special education is the greatest problem we have right now, and a large percentage of that is the inability of children to read because they have not been taught, and yet the cost of trying to bring them up to speed through tutors and so on can be very expensive. So any help that you can give us in that area, in a relatively inexpensive way, whether through software or relatively inexpensive equipment, would be a tremendous help to this country.

Mr. JADALLAH. Certainly, we have seen and I have read studies both around closed captioning, how kids just watching TV at home with closed captioning has actually helped increase their reading levels by capturing that television time. And certainly, we think utilizing the PC more helps them as well.

The computer is now part of literacy in the workplace, and it is really a core component. Much like reading and writing are a requirement in the workplace today, we are starting to see the same with computer literacy, the ability to use a PC, and that is something where we are absolutely committed to helping increase educational levels.

The CHAIRMAN. On the skill aspects, I have seen innovative programs—I think it is in Mississippi where they have modules where they are training people in high skill areas. Are you involved in producing those modules, or what are you doing in that area of helping individuals with higher-level skills?

Mr. JADALLAH. We are actually very excited. The IT, or information technology industry, right now in the United States has well over 300,000 open jobs. There is zero unemployment in this field, and if you have the right skills, you can get a very good-paying job.

The challenge is actually getting people to have those skills. It does not require a 4-year computer science degree at MIT in order to do well. In fact, we have launched a broad initiative that really helps people in under a year, sometimes in under 6 months, depending on their current skill level, to really come into the technology field. So they could be in other industries—we have some great examples of retired individuals who have basically become unretired. We also have other examples of individuals in the petroleum industry who have decided to come over, and ex-cab drivers who spend 6 months to a year learning the high-technology field and come in at great-paying jobs and really getting on the treadmill in a very positive way for them and for society.

The CHAIRMAN. How is that available? Is it through you, or through equipment you sell?

Mr. JADALLAH. Actually, that broad skills effort, the initiative that we call Skills 2000, we will be introducing a new component of that tomorrow through a partnership with an organization called Green Thumb. They work with the private industry councils, of which there are several hundred around the United States, and we are partnering with that organization, which is also, then, partnering in turn with Government funds, to help really educate and skill people into the information technology field.

They can come to our web site—microsoft.com/skills2000, or they can also call the Green Thumb organization, which is based here in the Washington area, for assistance,

The CHAIRMAN. Thank you very much.

Senator Harkin.

Senator HARKIN. This is very exciting and interesting. We have often thought of assistive technology just in terms of hardware, the devices that we use, and it is nice to know that you are also looking at the software, because the software has got to be equally accessible.

There are just two things I want to ask you about. You mentioned that you made some mistakes in your Explorer, that you had not built in Accessibility, and you went back to redo that. Is it Microsoft's policy now—I was looking at your five points—is it your policy now that before you come out with new versions of Office, for example, or NT or Windows, that you will have Accessibility built in? Is that a policy of Microsoft now?

Mr. JADALLAH. Yes. Essentially, as part of the five-point plan, we have got to really embrace Accessibility, heart and soul, inside the company, and part of that is a deep educational process with all of our developers to make sure they understand it and build it from the start, as opposed to worrying about it at the end. So it essentially is a policy. We will have that as part of Windows 98 and also the next release of Windows NT, and then on an ongoing basis.

Senator HARKIN. OK, so it is part of your policy. The second thing is that one of the problems is accessibility to the web. You mentioned "SAMI"?

Mr. JADALLAH. Yes. I actually did not mention the word, but Greg Lowney mentioned SAMI. It is a technical term, a code name—Synchronized—something.

Senator HARKIN. Could you tell me a little bit more about how that will work and when we can expect to see its emergence in the market, because I have talked with a lot of people with disabilities who want to access the web for one reason or another, and there is no software to do some of the things you are doing here with programs. I understand that SAMI is going to be able to do that; right?

Mr. JADALLAH. Exactly.

Senator HARKIN. So if I am going to put a home page on the web or something like that, I will probably have to do something, code it or something, so that SAMI can interpret it.

Mr. JADALLAH. Right; much in the same way that with television shows, in order to supply the closed captioning, you had to encode the closed captioning into the video signal.

Senator HARKIN. Line 17 or whatever.

Mr. JADALLAH. Yes, the vertical blanking or VBI signal. You will need to do something similar to that with the PC. Actually, the designer of SAMI is Dave Bolnick, so he can explain it.

Mr. BOLNICK. Basically, to make it easier for everyone to provide closed captioning, we separated out the caption content from the media. So that unlike TV, where you have to actually encode, and it is a very technical process, in our process, all you have to do is author, like you would author any document, a caption document, and this caption document is understood by our media player, and it synchronizes the two at the point of the user.

So the caption file can be on your web site, and it can be on someone else's web site. The media file can be on your web site, but in Germany, you may have a different caption file if it has German in it, and when they touch your web site, the two come together, and it is displayed according to the location. It is a very powerful approach, so it is separate and easy to author.

Senator HARKIN. Let me ask the question again. If I want to take my home page and make it accessible—when will SAMI be out? How soon will it be out?

Mr. BOLNICK. Next month.

Senator HARKIN. Will I have to do anything to my home page to make it accessible and interpretable by SAMI if someone is using that software?

Mr. BOLNICK. The way you would make your home page accessible for SAMI is that you would create a SAMI document, and you would request, just like you say you need to use Internet Explorer, you need to use Internet Explorer 4.0, because that is what SAMI is built into. And once that was in place, it would all work.

So that basically, you create your document, you request people to view this with——

Senator HARKIN. So I do not have to go back and redo the whole thing or anything like that?

Mr. BOLNICK. No.

Mr. JADALLAH. We would be glad to work with your staff on that as well.

Senator HARKIN. All right.

The CHAIRMAN. And mine.

Senator HARKIN. I am very intrigued by that. I think it is going to be a great device.

Mr. JADALLAH. I think that one of the key advantages that SAMI provides over previous methods is that it dramatically lowers the cost. In the past, you needed programmers and very technical, highly-paid people to encode and do the code and embed it into the file. And by having a clean separation, we can actually dramatically lower the cost of providing this captioning.

Mr. BOLNICK. We will be at the expo if you want a closer look at SAMI.

Mr. JADALLAH. Yes. We will be at the expo here, following this hearing, and if you would like to see it, we can show it to you.

Senator HARKIN. OK, thanks. I will see you there.

Thank you very much, Mr. Chairman.

The CHAIRMAN. Thank you all. That was extremely helpful, and we look forward to working with you. We understand the effort you are making, appreciate it and want to exploit it.

Mr. JADALLAH. Great. Thank you very much.

The CHAIRMAN. Thank you.

I will now call forward our second panel. Carol Smith is 21 years old and is a senior in regular education classes at the local high school in Knoxville, TN, local to Senator Bill Frist. Carol loves to give speeches, is in her school chorus and has her graduation in May. She hopes to attend Tennessee State Technical College and major in public speaking. She and her parents fought a long and courageous battle for her education. I am honored that she could be with us today to tell her story. Carol is joined by her mother, Jean.

Carol will also be joined by Corey L. Rowley, who is the chairperson of the Assistive Technology Task Force for the National Council on Independent Living. She has been active in assistive technology policy at the State and national level and now works closely with the Utah Assistive Technology Program to create a system in Utah that meets the needs of people with disabilities. We look forward to hearing about Utah's unique assistive technology program today.

We also welcome James Gashel, an individual whom I have known for many years, is director of government affairs for the National Federation of the Blind, a 50,000-member national organization of blind people. Previous to his current position, he worked for the Iowa Commission for the Blind and as a public school teacher in Minnesota. He has received a Commissioner's Award for Outstanding Leadership in Rehabilitation Services to the Disabled, as well as several other honors, for his work.

I look forward to hearing from him about the National Federation of the Blind's innovative programs in assistive technology.

I welcome all of you to this hearing. Why don't we start with Carol Smith.

STATEMENTS OF CAROL SMITH, STUDENT AND CONSUMER, KNOXVILLE, TN, ON BEHALF OF THE NATIONAL ASSOCIATION OF PROTECTION AND ADVOCACY SYSTEMS; COREY L. ROWLEY, LOGAN, UT, CHAIRPERSON, NATIONAL COUNCIL ON INDEPENDENT LIVING ASSISTIVE TECHNOLOGY TASK FORCE; AND JAMES GASHEL, BALTIMORE, MD, DIRECTOR OF GOVERNMENT AFFAIRS, NATIONAL FEDERATION OF THE BLIND

Ms. SMITH. Good morning, Chairman Jeffords, Senator Frist and members of the committee on Labor and Human Resources. My name is Carol Smith. I would like to tell you about myself and some of my experiences.

I live in Knoxville, TN with my parents, Billy and Jean Smith. I am 21 years old, and I have mixed cerebral palsy. When I was born, I had a breathing problem and had to stay in intensive care for 23 days. During that time, I had brain damage because my heart rate got so slow. At 16 months, the doctor told my parents I had cerebral palsy.

We lived in a rural area about 50 miles from Knoxville at the time. My parents drove me to Knoxville three times each week for me to get therapy. They wanted me to do the best I could for myself. I thank them for caring enough to do that.

I then started in the school system. They were supposed to provide my therapy and did some of the time. I was in a school for the disabled at that time. Since I cannot control my hands, I was told that I would not be able to operate a power wheelchair. I wanted to have some independence for myself.

In 1986, we learned of the University of Tennessee's Rehabilitation Engineering Program in Memphis. They designed a head control that allowed me to operate my chair myself. This was my first experience with technology to make my life better. That same year, I started in my first LRE classroom. LRE means least restrictive environment.

I did this to get in some time with the regular education students. I got to eat with them in the cafeteria and have interaction with my nondisabled peers. This was a great feeling for me. I made friends with a lot of them.

It was recommended that I get an Apple 2GS computer to use at school. The school system did not want to purchase it for me to use. My parents kept on insisting that I needed it until they finally got it for me. I used a head pointer to hit the keys on it. This was the latest technology at the time. I had to use the floppy disks back then to do my work. It was slow, but I worked hard to do my best. I went into the LRE program to be with regular students, but it did not offer much academics. I did not get much help or encouragement from my teacher.

Some people think that if you have cerebral palsy, you are retarded and cannot learn. I wanted to try some regular classes, but the school said no. I stayed in there for 7 years and was bored to tears.

Both of my parents are disabled, so we do not have much money. They felt so strongly about this that they took money they had saved and hired an attorney to get me out of there. This was before we learned of Tennessee Protection and Advocacy. The attorney told them that if they did not give me a chance, then they could not say I had failed.

I now have two teacher assistants that help me take notes. One helps in the morning, and the other in the evening. I use a motorized wheelchair to get around the campus of 1,400 students. I go to South Doyle High School in Knox County.

I have a communication device called Liberator. It is like the one that Bob Williams uses. I am in a speech class at school, and I use mine to do speeches. This is another example of how technology helps me.

I use a lot of technology in my life. It took a year to get the Liberator paid for. Tennessee Protection and Advocacy helped to get it funded. They operate the advocacy component of the Tech Act.

With the Liberator, I can hook it up to my computer and use it as my keyboard. I access it by using an infrared light like you use with your television. I can get on AOL and talk with my brother in California who is in the Navy. This saves a long-distance call to him. With the Liberator and my computer, I can get all kinds of information for my class work.

In the morning, my mom gets me up with more technology. She uses the Guildman overhead lifting system. It is electric, so it does all the work of lifting me out of bed and into the shower. She just guides it along a track. She can put me back in my chair then for school without having to life me. Mom has muscular dystrophy and does not have the strength to use a regular lift. This is a medical necessity for us, but the State's TennCare program has refused to pay for it. They say it is a luxury item.

This is the plan that replaced Medicaid in Tennessee. Tennessee Protection and Advocacy's assistive technology attorney, Lisa Terry, is helping us to get it paid for. She has gone above and beyond the call of duty to fight for me, and I appreciate it.

I have fought all my life to overcome my disability, only to be told by the TennCare medical director that maybe the best solution is to put me in a nursing home. They promised to pay for it until it was installed and then changed their minds. The total cost is $5,200 installed for the life. I ask you if it makes sense to pay hundreds of dollars per day for a nursing home when, with this lifting system, I can stay in my own home. I guess the Golden Rule is "He that has the gold makes the rules." I fail to see any wisdom in this at all.

I want you to please continue to fund the Tech Act to make sure that someone is there to help people like me to get the things that we need to survive in this world. Without assistive technology, we can only dream of participating in this game of life that we love so much. We need the advocacy that Tennessee Protection and Advocacy is providing. Sometimes their attorneys have to make the school system provide qualified therapists to work with people with communication devices or help people to get their services under TennCare or Medicare. I just want a level playing field to compete for my share of the American dream.

The Tech Act also helps to fund centers like the East Tennessee Technology Access Center in Knoxville. They did an evaluation on me to see what would work best for me. The disabled can go there to try computer switches and all kinds of devices before they buy them. This is really a valuable service to the disabled. Please help them keep up the good work. They also work with Tennessee Protection and Advocacy to protect the rights of people who cannot afford an attorney to fight for their technology needs. Your help is really needed to help them help others.

I think technology is wonderful. I know that in the future, new and better things will be available to help me. I also know that I will have to have the help of Tennessee Protection and Advocacy to help me get the things I have to have. I hope they will be there for me and for others like me.

I went to my senior prom last Saturday night with my boyfriend and had a great time. I want to go to college and maybe be a writer or a speaker. I would like to interview Barbara Walters sometime. I think she has integrity, and we need more women like her to serve as role models.

I can only answer yes and no questions right now. My parents can give you my answers if you want to ask me something. I want to say that this has been a great experience for a little girl from East Tennessee.

Please continue to fund the Tech Act so people like me can continue to fight for their independence and their dreams. I know you can make a difference for all of us.

Thanks for listening to me. Carol Smith.

[The prepared statement of Ms. Smith follows:]

PREPARED STATEMENT OF CAROL SMITH ON BEHALF OF THE NATIONAL ASSOCIATION OF PROTECTION AND ADVOCACY SYSTEMS (NAPAS)

Good morning Chairman Jeffords, Ranking Minority Member Kennedy, Senator Frist, and members of the Committee on Labor and Human Resources. My name is Carol Smith. I would like to thank members of the Committee on Labor and Human Resources for the opportunity to provide testimony on the reauthorization of the Technology-Related Assistance Act of 1988 (hereafter referred to as "the Tech Act").

The Personal Story of Carol Smith

I'd like to tell you about myself and some of my experiences. I live in Knoxville, Tennessee with my parents Billy and Jean Smith. I'm twenty-one years old and I have mixed cerebral palsy. When I was born, I had a breathing problem and had to stay in intensive care for twenty-three days. During that time, I experienced brain damage because my heart rate slowed down so much. When I was 16 months old, the doctor told my parents I had cerebral palsy. At that time we were living in a rural area about 50 miles from Knoxville. My parents drove me to Knoxville 3 times each week so I could receive therapy. I was experiencing speech and language delays and mobility problems related to both fine and gross motor skills. The therapy was recommended by the University of Tennessee's follow-up program and I received the services from the East Tennessee Children's Rehabilitation Program. I think these services were paid from through the state's Crippled Children's Program or Medicaid.

My parents wanted me to do the best I could for myself. I thank them for caring enough to want that for me. They continue to fight for my rights. My therapy continued until I reached the age of four. I then started in the school system where my therapy was supposed to continue. Although the school did provide my therapy, the provision of the therapy, which was recommended for one session a week, was inconsistent. I was in the school for the disabled at that time, that's where all children with disabilities went at that time.

Since I was unable to control my hands, I was told I wouldn't be able to operate a power wheelchair. I had been using a manual wheelchair since preschool and wanted a power wheelchair so I would have some independence for myself. In 1986, my parents and I learned of The University of Tennessee's Rehabilitation Engineering Program, located in Memphis. When I got my first power wheelchair two years ago, the staff at the Rehab Engineering Program designed a head control that allowed me to operate my chair by myself. This was my first experience with technology that could make my life better. That same year I started in my first LRE classroom. LRE means least restrictive environment. I was one of the first students in the Knox country public school system to be placed in a classroom with non-disabled students. I started in this classroom so that I could spend some time with the regular education students. I got to eat with them in the cafeteria and have interaction with my non-disabled peers. This was a great feeling for me. I made friends with a lot of these students.

It was recommended that I get an Apple 2GS computer to use at school. However, the school system did not want to purchase it for me because it was the school personnel's belief that I would not benefit from using a computer. My parents kept on insisting that I needed it, and they eventually got it for me. I used a head pointer to strike the keys on the computer. This was the latest technology at the time. I had to use the floppy disks back then to do my work. It was slow but I worked hard to do my best. I went into the LRE program to be with regular students but it didn't offer much academics. Although my teacher was a special education teacher, I did not get much help or encouragement from him. He seemed to think that all special education students were mentally retarded and would not benefit from academic studies. There was an aid in my class; however, my teacher and the aid were in constant conflict because my teacher thought the aid's desire to help kids was inappropriate. Although I wanted to try attending regular classes, the school continued to say no. As a result, I stayed in that special education classroom setting for 7 years and I was bored to tears.

Both of my parents are disabled so we don't have much money. They felt so strongly about this that they took money they had saved and hired an attorney to get me out of that school setting. This was before we learned of Tennessee Protection and Advocacy (P&A). The P&A attorney told the school personnel that if they didn't give me a chance then they couldn't say I had failed. The school agreed to let me try again with help. I now have 2 teacher's assistants that help me take notes. One helps in the morning and the other in the evening. I use a motorized wheelchair to get around the campus of 1400 students. I go to South Doyle High School in Knox County now and I am doing well.

When I was in my late teens, I applied to the state Vocational Rehabilitation (VR) agency for assistance in purchasing a communication device called a "Liberator." This devices is what Bob Williams, the recent Commissioner of the Administration on Developmental Disabilities, uses. VR denied funding for a Liberator, claiming that they did not believe that the Liberator would be used to assist me in employment. VR also noted that the purchase of a Liberator was not part of my transition plan.

Next we sought funding for the Liberator from TennCare. It took about a year to get funding for my Liberator and that was only after the Tennessee P&A assisted us in appealing a decision by TennCare to deny funding for a Liberator. Tennessee P&A operates the advocacy component of the Tech Act.

I can hook up my Liberator to my computer and use it as my keyboard. I access it by using an infrared light like you use with your television. I'm in a speech class at school and I use my Liberator to do my speeches. In addition, I can now access American on Line (AOL) and communicate with my brother who is in the Navy and stationed in California. This saves a long distance call to him. Using the Liberator and my computer, I can get all kinds of information for my class work. This is just one more example of how technology helps me. I use a lot of technology in my life.

In the mornings my Mom gets me up with more technology. She uses the Guildman overhead lifting system. It's electric so it does all the work of lifting me out of bed and into the shower. She just guides it along a track. She can put me back in my chair then for school without having to lift me. My parents used to lift me; however, my mom has muscular dystrophy and her doctor recently advised her to stop living me because her gross motor skills are unstable. Due to a recently diagnosed heart condition, my mom's doctor has advised her not to use a regular lift. Although this is a medical necessity for us, the state's TennCare program refuses to pay for the overhead lift. They said it was a luxury item. TennCare is the plan that replaced Medicaid in Tennessee. Tennessee P&A's Assistive Technology attorney, Alisa Terry, is helping us as we try to get the overhead lift paid for. In challenging TennCare's interpretation of "medical necessity" with regard to this AT device and TennCare's interpretation of state regulations, Ms. Terry has gone above and beyond the call of duty.

I really appreciate the help that I have received from Tennessee P&A. I have been fighting all of my life to overcome my disability, only to be told by the TennCare medical director that the best solution for me might be to put me in a nursing home. TennCare eventually agreed to pay for the lift; however, when it was installed and they found out it would cost a total of $5200, they decided not to pay for the lift. I ask you if it makes sense to pay hundreds of dollars per day for a nursing home when I can stay in my own home with this lifting system. I guess the Golden Rule to them is "he that has the gold makes the rules". I fail to see any wisdom in this at all.

I ask that you please continue to fund the Tech Act to make sure that someone is there to help people like me to get the equipment and services that we need to survive in this world. Without assistive technology we can only dream of participating in this game of life that we love so much. We need the advocacy that the Tennessee P&A is providing. Sometimes the P&A attorneys have to work with the school system to make them provide qualified therapists to work with people like me who use communication devices or with programs like Tenn Care or Medicare to get funding for the equipment and services that we need to increase our independence. I just want a level playing field to compete for my share of the American dream.

The Tech Act also helps to fund centers like the East Tennessee Technology Access Center in Knoxville. They did an evaluation on me to see what would work best for me. Individuals with disabilities can go there to try computer switches and other kinds of devices before they purchase them. This is really a valuable service for individuals with disabilities. Please help them keep up the good work. They also work with Tennessee P&A to protect the rights of people that can't afford an attorney to fight for their technology needs. Your help is really needed to help them help others.

I think technology is wonderful. I know in the future that new and better things will be available to help me. I am sure I will need the assistance of the Tennessee P&A to help me get the things I need to function more independently. I hope they'll be there for me and others like me.

I went to my Senior Prom last Saturday night with my boyfriend and I had a great time. I want to go to college and maybe be a writer or speaker. I'd like to interview Barbara Walters sometime. I think she has integrity and we need more women like her to serve as role models.

I can only answer yes and no questions right now. My parents can assist me with answers if you want to ask me something else about my life. I want to say that this has been a great experience for a little girl from East Tennessee. Please continue to fund the Tech Act, and particularly the P&A program in the Tech Act, so that people like me can continue to fight for their independence and their dreams. I know you can make a difference for all of us.

Thanks for listening to me and I hope you will refer to the written testimony that I am submitting on behalf of myself and the National Association of Protection and Advocacy Systems (NAPAS) for additional information on the important role that protection and advocacy services can have for individuals with disabilities who are having difficulty obtaining the assistive technology equipment and services that they need to increase their independence and productivity.

The National Association of Protection and Advocacy Systems (NAPAS)

NAPAS is a national, nonprofit membership organization comprised of federally-funded Protection and Advocacy (P&A) Programs and the Client Assistance Program (CAP). These programs, which are conducted in each state and territory, are authorized to pursue legal, administrative and other appropriate remedies to protect the rights of all individuals with disabilities. They also advocate on behalf of such individuals to ensure that they have access to needed services and supports, including access to educational services, employment and training services, Social Security benefits and medical care, public transportation, housing, etc. Further, P&As, in particular, devote considerable resources to ensure access for people with disabilities to the assistive technology (AT) devices and services that can be the most critical factor in facilitating such individuals* ability to fully participate in all aspects of life. NAPAS and its member programs are committed to ensuring the self-determination, independence, empowerment, integration and inclusion of children and adults with disabilities into all aspects of American society.

NAPAS recognizes the important role that AT can have in the lives of people with disabilities. Without appropriate and affordable AT devices and services, many individuals with disabilities are unable to maximize their independence, abilities, capacities, contributions, productivity and ability to learn, work and play in all life settings. For many individuals with disabilities, the provision of AT devices and services is the most critical factor in expanding their abilities and circumventing the functional limitations of their disabilities. Moreover, if the vision behind the passage of the Americans with Disabilities Act is ever to be fully realized, individuals with disabilities must have access to a wide range of appropriate and affordable AT.

Throughout the 1980s, specific references to AT were inserted into a variety of disability laws, including the Rehabilitation Act, the Individuals with Disabilities Education Act (IDEA), and the Older Americans Act. However, it was not until 1988 that the first comprehensive AT legislation was passed by Congress. With the passage of the Tech Act, Congress recognized the potential of AT as a means of achieving equal access and expanding opportunities for individuals with disabilities. For the last ten years, the activities funded under the Tech Act have greatly impacted the availability and quality of AT devices and services, and have facilitated much progress in this area.

The Tech Act provides discretionary grants to the states and territories to assist them in developing and implementing consumer-responsive, comprehensive statewide programs of technology-related assistance for individuals with disabilities of all ages. In order to receive funding under Title I of the Tech Act, the Governor of a state or territory must designate a lead agency which is responsible for:

• coordinating efforts related to, and supervising the preparation and submission of, the application for funding;

• administering and supervising the use of the funds awarded to the state/territory;

• coordinating the planning, development, implementation, and evaluation of the consumer-responsive, comprehensive, statewide program of technology-related assistance among public agencies and between public agencies and private agencies, including coordinating efforts related to entering into interagency agreements; and

• coordinating efforts related to, and supervising the active, timely, and meaningful participation by individuals with disabilities and their representatives, and other interested individuals, with respect to activities carried out under the grant.

The Tech Act also requires these lead agencies (hereafter referred to as *Tech Act Project or TAP*) to examine barriers to accessing and using AT in their respective states/territories and then to work to eliminate these barriers permanently. Over the first eight years of funding, the TAPs have focused on overcoming barriers in three major areas: access to AT, availability of AT, and funding for AT.

When the Tech Act was originally conceptualized, it was viewed as a time-limited source of financial assistance to support systems change and advocacy activities on the state level to "increase the availability of funding for, access to, and provision of," AT devices and services. As a result, Title I was drafted to sunset in 1999. The programs and activities authorized for funding under Title I were very broad in scope, with most activities being permissive rather than mandatory. Consequently, the activities undertaken by the TAPs are many and varied. The list of activities undertaken covers the gamut from informing people about the availability and capabilities of AT to actually assisting individuals in acquiring needed AT. While being given such broad authorities, the TAPs were subjected to only minimal accountability.

Early in the implementation of the Tech Act it became evident that many individuals with disabilities would need individualized advocacy services and, on occasion, legal representation in order to effectively challenge Medicaid, Medicare, the school system, and/or private insurance companies when they are being denied access to the AT devices and services that they need. Consequently, when Congress reauthorized the Tech Act in 1994, Section 101(b)(20) mandated that each TAP use a portion of its Title I funding to make a grant or enter into a contract with an entity to support protection and advocacy (P&A) services through the systems established to provide P&A services under the Developmental Disabilities Assistance and Bill of Rights Act. Under Section 101(f), the P&As are directed to use the funding made available through these grants/contracts to provide legally-based protection and advocacy services for individuals with disabilities with regard to their AT needs. This advocacy component of the TAPs is known as the Protection and Advocacy for Assistive Technology (PAAT) Program. Grants to the P&A systems in the states/territories generally ranged from $40,000 to $100,000 annually.

Similar to the TAPs, the PAAT Projects are mandated to conduct activities that are consumer-responsive and that will result in increased access to funding for AT devices and services. They are authorized to undertake legal, administrative and other appropriate means of representation to implement systems change and advocacy services. They are also instructed to develop and implement strategies designed specifically to enhance the long-term abilities of individuals with disabilities and their family members or representatives to successfully advocate for AT devices and services for which such individuals may be eligible under other laws. In addition, P&As are responsible for coordinating with protection and advocacy services funded through other sources and coordinating activities with the systems change and advocacy activities carried out by the State lead agency for the TAP. Moreover, P&As are responsible for undertaking individual, group, and systemic advocacy to facilitate the access that individuals with disabilities have to AT devices and services.

PAAT Projects Are Successfully Advocating for AT Devices and Services

The PAAT Projects have been very successful in undertaking individual advocacy with regard to AT issues. Most of the state P&A systems report that they:

• have experienced a significant change in their ability to respond to AT issues as a result of their contracts with the TAPs;

• now include AT among their annual priorities (i.e., approximately 87 percent report this);

• are now able to dedicate staff to AT issues or set up a new speciality unit to deal with AT issues;

• have used PAAT funding to provide cross-programmatic training on AT issues, providing P&A staff across all programs with a greater awareness of AT and an enhanced competence on AT issues;

• have staff with an enhanced ability to spot and deal with AT issues as they undertake issue identification and develop appropriate service plans;

• are able to represent many more individuals with disabilities as they seek access to AT devices and services; and

• have been able to expand their public education campaigns, and their training and outreach activities to educate consumers and others about AT issues and the P&A's ability to provide individual case advocacy with regard to AT issues.

PAAT Projects nationwide have represented thousands of individuals with disabilities in their efforts to obtain AT devices and services from federally-funded programs such as Special Education and Vocational Rehabilitation, and from federal funding sources such as Medicaid and Medicare. PAAT Projects have also been successful in representing individuals with disabilities in their attempts to secure funding for AT devices and services from private insurance companies. The successes of the PAAT Projects are the result of a variety of advocacy activities. For example, the Wisconsin PAAT Project has worked with 323 individuals during the last five years. Ninety-seven (97) of those individuals received individualized advocacy services and 225 received information and referral services. During each of those five years, the Wisconsin PAAT Program was involved in approximately 15 in-depth consultations on cases with other advocates who were also working with individuals with disabilities on AT issues. In addition, the Wisconsin PAAT Project provided training to an average of 300 people per year. Such training is often used to teach people about their rights under various laws and to instruct them on how to self advocate.

An example of individual case advocacy provided by the Wisconsin PAAT Project involved an 8 year old boy who nearly drowned. The boy suffered from anoxia, which resulted in a temporary comatose state and permanent brain damage. His family and therapist applied to Medicaid for a piece of durable medical equipment (a stander) to provide home physical therapy to the boy. The boy required the stander to assist him with standing and to benefit his overall physical functioning, e.g., his circulation, respiration, bone density, kidney functioning, etc. Medicaid denied the stander on the basis that the boy was not cognitively or developmentally capable of benefiting from the traditional use of a stander. Advocates from the Wisconsin PAAT Project represented the boy in a fair hearing. The Hearing Officer decided on behalf of the boy, stating that the overall medical need established at the hearing necessitated the purchase of the stander by Wisconsin Medicaid. A recent call from the boy's family indicated that the boy was able to respond more actively to family communications and he is exceeding the expectations of his physicians and care givers. He will be going back to school in the fall.

In another situation, the Wisconsin PAAT Project represented a 13 year old girl who is dependent on a ventilator and has severe medical complications which prevent her from attending school. She is in the 6th grade through a home bound instruction program. The PAAT project assisted her with obtaining internet access for community interaction, the ability to explore her world and to communicate with her classmates at school via an e-mail pen pal program. The girl is now able to do classroom presentations and participate in on-line events at school.

The NY PAAT Project provided technical assistance to a woman who was denied approval by her private insurance company for a stand-up wheelchair. The woman was in need of the therapeutic benefits of standing which can often, by increasing the blood flow, prevent additional medical problems from developing. A stand-up chair also allows its user to lead a more independent life, giving the person the ability to reach items within the kitchen or bathroom that could not be reached from a seated position. When the woman, who lives 270 miles from the PAAT office, sought assistance from the NY PAAT Project, she was provided with extensive technical assistance by phone. As a result, the woman was able to self-advocate and write her own very compelling appeal letter to the insurance company. The insurance company reversed its decision and approved the funding necessary for the standing wheelchair.

The Hawaii P&A provides another example of the success that a PAAT Project can have in getting individuals with disabilities the AT devices and services that they need. During one ten month period, the HI P&A used PAAT funding to provide individualized advocacy which resulted in six individuals obtaining wheelchairs; two individuals obtaining augmentative communication devices; one individual obtaining a shower chair; and one individual getting an electric lift. The HI P&A reports that it has found legally-based intervention by the P&A to be one of the most effective means of getting its State Departments of Education, Medicaid, Medicare and Vocational Rehabilitation to provide AT devices and services for their clients.

P&As nationwide also report substantial success in advocating for the needs of groups of individuals with disabilities. In many states, individual case advocacy on the part of the P&A has resulted in systemic changes, e.g., changes in rules, regulations, policies, procedures and/or state laws, which ultimately benefits large numbers of individuals with disabilities with similar AT needs. For example, one state reported that the P&A's advocacy efforts resulted in changes to the fair hearing processes, causing state Medicaid agencies to establish policies which recognize that specific AT devices can be funded by Medicaid. In another state, PAAT litigation established and clarified criteria to allow specific AT devices to be funded under Medicaid. PAAT activities in another state resulted in new policies being established which designated funding for the rental of AT devices. Another PAAT program was instrumental in getting state policies modified to ensure that AT was approved as a fundable item in specific waiver programs.

A specific example of individual case advocacy resulting in systemic change involves a young man who is being represented by the Wisconsin PAAT Project. The young man has cerebral palsy, is nonverbal, and can only communicate *yes* and *no* by nodding his head. He uses a wheelchair and has some vision problems as well. Although his receptive language skills far exceed his expressive language skills, his inability to communicate made an accurate assessment of his cognitive functioning impossible. When a communication device that met his needs was prescribed, trial uses at home and in the community provided him with the ability to communicate with relatives and friends as never before. Based on these trials, a Dynavox augmentative communication device, which costs $5,000, was prescribed for this young man, along with a wheelchair mount for mounting the device, a "Buddy Switch" for turning the device on and off, and a color monitor so he would be better able to see the options on the device.

When state Medicaid received a request for prior authorization for this communication system, approval was granted for only $5,000 based on a Wisconsin Medicaid policy implemented years ago. The policy limits Medicaid funding to no more than $5,000 per ten year life expectancy for a communication device. Acknowledging that the young man needed the complete system, Medicaid maintained that the young man and his family would have to seek additional funding elsewhere for the special components he needed. The Wisconsin PAAT Project challenged this policy in circuit court, arguing that the policy was arbitrary and capricious and that it did not meet the medical needs of people like this young man. The circuit court struck down the policy.

There are many other examples of PAAT Projects undertaking individual case advocacy that ultimately resulted in systemic change. For example, two states have reported that they were able to get power wheelchairs for individuals in nursing homes. Six states report that the PAAT Program was instrumental in getting augmentative communication devices funded for adults and children with disabilities who were in need of such devices.

The list of AT devices and services obtained by individuals who benefited from PAAT assistance is probably as long and diverse as the needs of different people with different types of disabilities. Some individuals have obtained computer equipment or adaptations for computer equipment. Others have obtained various types of lifts, replacement wheelchairs, access ramps, hearing aids, and other types of equipment and devices. As a result, many, many individuals now experience a new or renewed level of independence.

On occasion, the P&A may find it necessary to resort to more formal means of resolving disputes, e.g., formal appeals or litigation. For example, in the Matter of Starkweather v. Wing (N.Y. Appellate Division, 4th Dept. 1997), the New York PAAT represented a 14 year old boy who lived with his grandparents and who was seeking funding for a customized power wheelchair. Both grandparents had major back problems and their ability to care for their grandson was compromised without the power wheelchair, putting this child in danger of being institutionalized. The court approved the funding, reasoning that the power wheelchair was needed to increase the independence and functional ability of the boy, especially in emergency situations, and to prevent the development of "learned helplessness."

With regard to special education students, numerous PAAT Programs report that an increased awareness of AT issues is being seen within both State Education Agencies (SEAs) and Local Education Agencies (LEAs). Teachers and education officials are more aware of how AT can assist students and are, therefore, more willing to provide AT devices and services. Other states report that LEAs are better able to access Medicaid to fund AT now that P&As are investing resources in providing training on AT issues. As a result, more children are receiving AT as the funding burden has been reallocated away from the schools.

With regard to students with disabilities who are transitioning from special education to vocational rehabilitation services, the PAAT program in one state facilitated the development of an agreement between state agencies regarding a specific provision in a state law allowing AT purchased with special education money to stay with the child as a VR service after the child leaves school and seeks VR services. In another state, the PAAT Program was able to get the State VR agency to acknowledge that, under federal law, when AT is involved there is no requirement to exhaust other funding sources before VR agency money is used. In one state, PAAT Project staff were successful in getting the State VR agency to establish procedures that would ensure that AT needs were reviewed as individuals were developing their individualized written rehabilitation programs. One PAAT Program worked in collaboration with the State VR agency to influence the state to implement better bidding procedures for vendors which eliminated unnecessary delays in obtaining AT devices.

The PAAT Projects have been involved in many other efforts to modify laws and policies. In a few states, PAAT has worked to see that polling places have the assistive technology necessary to ensure access for individuals with disabilities. In several states, PAAT has worked in collaboration with other groups to see that AT Lemon Laws are passed, i.e., consumer protection legislation for AT items like electric wheelchairs. Several PAAT Projects have worked to see that hospitals establish policies to provide AT to meet the needs of patients who are deaf. In many cases, PAAT representatives have worked collaboratively with the TAPs to accomplish these important systemic changes.

While strongly supporting the litigation component of the P&A program, NAPAS believes that the use of non-attorney advocates and paralegals is a cost-effective use of the limited budgets available for these programs, particularly the modest statewide budgets being awarded for the P&A component of the TAPs. The use of advocates and paralegals is also efficient and cost-effective, given that a substantial percentage of a typical P&A's caseload consists of informal advocacy and administrative hearings where an attorney is not required. Moreover, P&As resolve disputes using lower level resolution strategies (e.g., consultation, conciliation, negotiation, mediation and other forms of alternative dispute resolution) whenever possible.

Recommendations Regarding the Current Reauthorization

NAPAS staff worked with staff from Senator Jeffords' office as S. 1579, the Rehabilitation Act Amendments of 1998, was being drafted. This bipartisan piece of legislation was drafted with substantial input from the disability community, including individuals with disabilities and their advocates, public and private service providers, and other interested parties. S. 1579 constitutes a major rewrite of key sections of the Rehab Act. For example, the 36 State plan requirements in Section 101 were consolidated and streamlined into 24 requirements in S. 1579. This and other provisions are intended to simplify the administration of the program. In addition, the amended Rehab Act places greater emphasis on interagency cooperation and coordination, including spelling out a dispute resolution process to use when interagency disputes arise. Concepts such as consumer choice and empowerment are enhanced. Due process requirements and accountability measures are strengthened in S. 1579. Certain terms and phrases which are used extensively in disability legislation are defined in the amended Rehab Act for the purposes of creating consistency across disability programs and reducing legislative text.

NAPAS recommends that a similar effort be undertaken in the reauthorization of the Tech Act. The bill should be thoroughly reviewed to find ways to simplify language and use terminology that is consistent with terminology in other disability legislation.

NAPAS believes that the current reauthorization is the appropriate vehicle to revisit the time-limited nature of the Tech Act. If funding under the Tech Act sunsets in 1999 as originally proposed, only nine of the 56 states and territories will have benefited from the full ten-year funding cycle authorized for the TAPs. Considering the significant changes in our society over the last ten years (e.g., welfare reform, movement toward managed care, efforts to block grant federally-funded employment and training programs, etc.) and the continuation of major breakthroughs in technology (e.g., in terms of availability, user friendliness, and reduced costs), the time-limited nature of the federal assistance available under the Tech Act seems inappropriate. Indeed, advances in technology and changes in programmatic authorities and funding streams are more likely to increase the need for the continuation of federal support to the states and territories to ensure that individuals with disabilities can obtain and effectively utilize AT devices and services.

NAPAS recommends that the Tech Act be reauthorized to continue to provide federal support to the states and territories in their efforts to increase the access that individuals with disabilities have to appropriate and affordable AT devices and services. As the amendments to the Tech Act are drafted, Congressional staff should take a close look at the long list of permissive authorities in current law in an effort to eliminate some authorities and combine and streamline others to develop a more targeted list of authorized activities. NAPAS recommends that continuation funding under Title I be appropriated for three specific categories of activities:

1) continuation funding for the TAPs currently authorized under Title I to ensure that a ten-year cycle is completed in each state and territory;

2) for those states and territories completing their ten-year TAP cycle, the re-directing of Title I funding to be awarded on a competitive grant basis to programs and projects that have demonstrated their ability to increase the access that individuals with disabilities have to the AT devices and services that they needs; and

3) the establishment of a separate authorization available through direct funding to the P&A system in each state and territory for the provision of legal, administrative and other appropriate remedies to ensure access to AT devices and services.

1) *Completion of a Ten-Year Cycle for Each Tech Act Projects*

NAPAS recommends that funding continue to be available to all TAPs for the full ten-year grant period authorized in the original Tech Act. As the TAPs in the individual states and territories complete this ten-year cycle, Tech Act funds should continue to be available to these states; however, the use of these funds should be more targeted.

2) *States with Targeted Funding*

For those states and territories that have completed their ten-year TAP cycle, NAPAS recommends that funds continue to be available to these states or territories for distribution through a competitive grant process. The activities authorized for this funding should be more targeted than under current law, i.e., being targeted for programs and projects that have demonstrated the ability to increase the number of individuals who actually obtain and can effectively use AT services and devices. NAPAS recommends that the focus of funding activities be shifted from those with the primary purpose of increasing knowledge of AT options to those which actually facilitate access to needed services and devices, e.g., equipment loan/recycling programs, the establishment and continuation of demonstration/evaluation centers, the creation of financial loan programs, the creation of state policies such as lemon laws, etc. NAPAS believes that funding available for information, education and referral services should be limited and that, to the maximum extent possible, greater emphasis should be placed on the utilization of existing resources for the provision of such services, e.g., existing web sites, ABLEDATA, etc.

In many states, the establishment of programs that provide for the recycling of AT or that establish opportunities for AT devices to be obtained on loan have proven to be effective in increasing the access that individuals with disabilities have to AT devices. Although most of the states have already undertaken some type of recycling effort under current law, a model program has not emerged yet due to the complicated nature of certain issues that must be addressed (e.g., confidentiality, liability, solicitation, etc.).

Consumer services and technical assistance were not mentioned in the 1992 amendments to the Tech Act; nevertheless, many states have tried to do something with Title I funds to address this critical need. Some people believe that the ability to provide consumer services and technical assistance could potentially be of greater benefit to individuals with disabilities than almost any other provision that might be in the amended Tech Act. Hence, programs providing technical assistance and technical support will continue to be needed, as will programs providing appropriate evaluations and training in the use and maintenance of AT devices. Federal support must continue to be available to assist in facilitating a network of essential technical services to help consumers make better utilization of the technology they obtain. Consumers will continue to need assistance in setting up AT equipment and devices, training on how to use the AT, and instructions on troubleshooting, problem solving, and the maintenance of existing AT equipment and devices.

NAPAS recommends that the activities authorized under Title I include assistance in establishing technical support systems which provide access to experienced people who will provide maintenance and repair services in a person's home when necessary. Funds should also be authorized to support projects that refurbish or tune-up equipment or that facilitate reutilization or recycling networks. Programs and projects of technical assistance and support should be required to coordinate with programs that recycle AT equipment and devices and/or that are involved in the sales and/or loan of equipment. Technical assistance and technical support will also be necessary to ensure an adequate understanding of safety and liability issues. Among other things, the availability of appropriate technical assistance and support should help to alleviate the high incidence of AT abandonment and down time.

NAPAS also recommends that authorized activities be targeted toward the identification and removal of barriers which restrict or limit access to AT. For example, NAPAS recommends that Title I discretionary funding be targeted for programs and projects that promote interagency cooperation and coordination and that will ensure a widespread understanding of the needs of individuals with disabilities with regard to AT devices and services. A great deal of work remains to be done to facilitate coordination between state disability service agencies and to identify and remove barriers created by federal and state laws, regulations and policies. For example, recycling and equipment loan programs will only be effective if policies can be changed to ensure that AT funding programs such as private insurance, health, and vocational rehabilitation will authorize the purchase of used equipment when it is appropriate for the individual. Likewise, established policies in many states still need to be modified to provide reimbursement for AT professional services provided by occupational therapists, physical therapists, speech and language therapists, and engineers.

Critical Criteria for Awarding Competitive Grants: If designated funds allotted to the states and territories under Title I of the Tech Act are to be distributed through a competitive grant process, the Act should spell out the primary selection criteria to be used in evaluating applications for funding. Such criteria should include, at a minimum, an applicant's ability to:

- simplify and enhance access to AT devices and services;
- ensure the creation of a consumer responsive program or project;
- maintain independence from programs and projects that provide funding for AT or set reimbursement policies for AT;
- provide easy access to information technology;
- demonstrate meaningful involvement in interagency cooperation, collaboration, and coordination on the state and local levels;
- create strong linkages with the state P&A systems and with other public and private programs and projects that provide services to individuals with disabilities on the local, state, regional and national levels.

3) *Continued Financial Support for Protection and Advocacy Services*

NAPAS recommends that a portion of the funds appropriated under Title I of the Tech Act be reserved for distribution to the protection and advocacy systems authorized under the Developmental Disabilities Assistance and Bill of Rights Act to support the continuation of legally-based advocacy services for individuals with disabilities who are seeking to access to AT devices and services. NAPAS believes that the availability of legally-based advocacy must continue to ensure that the rights of individuals with disabilities are protected.

The P&As have been instrumental in ensuring the individuals with disabilities have had access to appropriate AT devices and services, and in many cases, have been able to use their individual advocacy efforts to facilitate systemic change. Given current changes resulting from welfare reform, the implementation of managed care, and rapidly expanding communications and transportation technologies, the need for individualized and group advocacy could potentially increase substantially in the next two to three years. The availability of P&A services will play a critical role in ensuring that individuals with disabilities have access to the AT devices and services that they need to fully participate in society, including ensuring access to appropriate evaluations and being available to assist individuals with disabilities to fully participate in the planning of their lives. For example, many disputes will arise in the upcoming years over eligibility for AT devices and services under new health and welfare laws, regulations, and policies. P&A will also need to continue their efforts to monitor rapid expansions in communications and transportation technology to ensure that individuals with disabilities will be included in the planning and development of systems and that they will have access once the systems are in place. Moreover, individuals with disabilities, particularly individuals with the most severe disabilities, will continue to need access to advocacy services, and, on occasion, legal representation in order to obtain appropriate AT evaluations and to secure access to and funding for AT devices and services.

With regard to the funding available for the provision of protection and advocacy services, NAPAS recommends that a percentage of the total funding available under Title I of the Tech Act be set aside to be distributed to the P&A systems in the states and territories on a formula grant basis. A minimum allotment should be established for the provision of P&A services to ensure that each state and territory has adequate funding to ensure effective implementation of the P&A component of the Tech Act.

Direct Funding for P&A Activities: NAPAS recommends that financial support for the continuation of the protection and advocacy component of the Tech Act be awarded directly to the P&A system. If Congress does reauthorize the Tech Act to provide additional funding to the states and territories that have completed their ten-year cycle and such funding is to be distributed among programs within the states/territories on a competitive grant basis, such direct funding would be necessary since there would no longer be a lead agency in the state/territory and since multiple grants would likely be awarded in many states and territories. In addition, direct funding would eliminate some of the inappropriate disputes that have emerged in several states as the PAAT contracts were being negotiated between the lead agency for the TAP and the P&A system. The contracting process has sometimes been used improperly limit the P&As exercise of its legitimate authorities.

For example, in a recent negotiation between the TAP and the P&A, the TAP sought to impose restrictions on the activities that could be undertaken with the PAAT funding. The TAP asked the P&A to refrain from advocating for systemic change without first having an individual client. Such a restriction appears to be in direct violation of the intent of the Act as currently written and would be extremely inefficient if the P&A was made aware of a systemic problem through a source other than individual case advocacy. Since similar issues have arisen in other states and territories around the negotiation of the PAAT contracts, it seems obvious that this approach to funding for P&A services often poses a conflict of interest.

In some instances, other types of conflicts have arisen as a result of the existing relationship between the P&A and the state agency designated to serve as the lead agency for the TAP. For example, in many states, the designated lead agency is the State Vocational Rehabilitation (VR) Agency. If the P&A houses the Client Assistance Program (CAP) and the CAP has been aggressive in ensuring the rights of individuals seeking or receiving vocational rehabilitation services from the State VR Agency, the relationship between these two agencies could already be strained. Since many of the programs that provide funding for AT devices and services are housed in state agencies, the idea of providing funding to state agencies that are service providers to be used in advocating for the provision of AT devices and services seems inappropriate.

Appropriating Funding for Title III

Although Title III of the 1994 amendments to the Tech Act provided for model funding programs, no funds have been appropriated for these provisions to date. Congress should either appropriate funds for this purpose or introduce new legislation which will stimulate model assistive technology funding efforts, e.g., interest-free loans, direct grants, private and state financial partnerships, small-end grants, and model programs that would help consumers navigate the AT funding maze. Moreover, NAPAS recommends that funding continue to be available for national projects addressing technical assistance, training, technology transfer and recycling, business opportunities for individuals with disabilities, and alternative financing for devices and services.

Summary

In summary, NAPAS recommends that greater emphasis be placed in Title I on funding activities that result in measurable outcomes, e.g., the actual acquisition of assistive technology for individuals with disabilities. In addition, NAPAS recommends that Federal initiatives be established to promote universal design, i.e., the idea that all equipment and services should be designed for use by the largest percentage of the population, including individuals with disabilities.

Over the next few weeks, NAPAS will continue to work with representatives from the PAAT Projects, with representatives from the Consortium for Citizens with Disabilities (CCD), and with other interested parties to further expand on the recommendations for the reauthorization of the Tech Act. NAPAS looks forward to working with congressional and Committee staff as the reauthorized bill is being drafted and marked up. Please feel free to contact Curt Decker or Sallie Rhodes at NAPAS if you have any questions about the information or recommendations in this testimony.

The CHAIRMAN. Thank you, Carol. That was wonderful. I have never been so moved and so thankful that we have developed the kind of technology that has opened your eyes and made it possible for you to live in our society in a meaningful way. Your smile has made my heart smile.

I do have a couple of questions for you. Has your use of technology in school had a positive effect on your teachers and classmates?

Ms. SMITH. Yes.

The CHAIRMAN. Thank you so much. And how has it impacted you in regard to your teachers—do they now give you more challenging assignments to do?

Ms. SMITH. Yes.

The CHAIRMAN. Well, thank you so much, Carol. You have made all of our lives a little bit better today, and we just hope the best for you as you go on to college and whatever your life may bring to you. Thank you so much for being here.

Ms. SMITH. You are welcome.

The CHAIRMAN. Ms. Rowley, please proceed.

Ms. ROWLEY. Senator Jeffords, I appreciate being invited to testify today on the needs for assistive technology. I was asked to discuss two things, the first being as chairman of the Assistive Technology Task Force for the National Council on Independent Living, to talk about some of the things that our organization believes should belong in a new Tech Act or technology-related bill; and the second, being that I work very closely with the Utah Assistive Technology Program, I have been asked to discuss some of the things that have led to the successes that we have had there and maybe some steps that would work in a general way.

I became involved in the national discussion about technology legislation when I approached the governing board of the National Council on Independent Living about the Tech Act. I was very surprised at their reaction, because although assistive technology is a critical issue for centers for independent living, many were not working with their State tech projects even though the focus for systems change in the Tech Act and the advocacy role of independent living centers creates a natural partnership. I was surprised at this, because I have been active with the efforts in Utah, and we were very anxious to see this continue.

The Utah Assistive Technology Program, which is funded by the Tech Act, has been in existence for 9 years. It has reached a point in our State where we are able to look back and evaluate some of the steps that we have taken to create permanent systems change in Utah's program.

As I went through and talked with the director of the project—and I should make it clear that I do not work for the project; I work with independent living, but we have worked very closely to ensure that consumer perspective was brought and that the consumers were determining what needed to happen—so we went back and looked at the things that we have done and that our State has done and that the project has coordinated to help us believe that what we have is a very effective assistive technology system within our State.

The first factor that we found to be very critical was that the project was not placed within a State agency. The Tech Act originally called for changes to be made in education, Medicaid and the vocational rehabilitation programs and their assistive technology policies. In my opinion, the effectiveness of the project and the ability to make those changes is compromised when you work for that system. In Utah's case, the tech project is in a university-affiliated program which is independent of the State service system.

The second thing that happened in our State was that representation from each State agency that provided services to people with disabilities is required to be on the management and implementation board. That board is the governing body for the tech program, and in almost every situation, members of that board are the directors of agencies such as Medicaid, Health and Human Services, and

Voc Rehab. Those directors sit on the board, and they are not substitutes without decisionmaking authority. So that when the M and I board discusses a better way to get coverage for equipment from Medicaid, the Medicaid director is there to respond or feel the pressure so they understand what the consumers require.

It is important to note that the Utah Assistance Technology Program staff are staff to the board, not staff to the agencies.

A Utah Assistive Technology Program Consumer Council was established. This is where I think we have had a lot of success. All of the Consumer Council members are either persons with disabilities or parent advocates. The consumers get together, and they identify barriers surrounding assistive technology. Most of them are users of technology, and they have a real discussion about the barriers in our State. That is when they are meeting as their own board. They have this discussion and identify the problems and barriers, and they then report these issues to the M and I board. The board is required to respond in writing on activities that they have undertaken to take care of these barriers.

I think what has really pushed the success is that the Consumer Council meets individually to identify these barriers, but they also join this management board as full members with equal voting rights. So that—for instance, I will go back to the Medicaid discussion—if the barrier has been identified to getting a communication device through Medicaid, if the consumer is not a member of this board, the director could say we handle that, provide that in writing, and it would go on. But now we have created a peer situation, because the consumer has the same voting right as that Medicaid director, and there is really good discussion that goes on between them, and it brings them together.

I should also point out that the bylaws of the management board State that the Consumer Council has veto rights over any action of the board. So if they get together as a group and decide that a policy is not right, they can veto it at any time.

Another element of the Utah project is that each initiative is required to be sustainable. We felt like that was a focus in the legislation that you put forward—that is, systems were changed, and they would be permanent, that even when the Tech Act was due to sunset, the gains that had been achieved would still be in place.

As each barrier was identified and worked on, the project kept in mind that it was time-limited. Not only did the project need to address the barrier but to plan how the solution would continue after the tech program was gone. As a result, the sustainability activities focused on State funding, policy changes, and State legislative changes. Tech Act dollars were spent on each initiative with a clear understanding that when continuing support was found, the funds from the project would cease.

It is important to note that the responsibility for sustainability remained with the project and was not passed on to the subcontractors. In many instances, a tech project would give a contract to an assistive technology service entity with the expectation that when the contract ends, the entity would be able to sustain or maintain the program. Often, that is written into the contract. While this may sound good, the entity often does not have the capacity to find other resources to support it. Even though the subcontractor can be part of the answer, I believe that the responsibility to provide resources and coordination should be left with the Tech Act project.

Hand-in-hand with sustainability are efforts to build capacity. That is also something that you talked about in your legislation. To build capacity, you have to utilize an ongoing community resource. As you change a program's assistive technology capabilities, you integrate technology into the services that are already being provided. The exciting thing about that is that when a consumer or someone with a disability needs assistive technology services, he can go to the place where he is already receiving services. If you build up the capacity of the vocational rehabilitation system, then, as a consumer looking for employment, you cannot look at assistive technology in its own space, so those come together—the counselor who is helping to find employment can understand and help them achieve their goals with technology. It just creates a natural partnership that does not make a consumer or person with a disability have to go elsewhere and find assistive technology in its own arena.

In Utah, this has happened in our centers for independent living, as one of the examples I would like to tell you about. The Tech Act and the Utah Office of Rehabilitation developed a system of assistive technology coordinators. They place coordinators around the State, within the centers—and I wish Senator Harkin were here, because we do understand the rural issue, and we have worked on it extensively. These assistive technology coordinators conduct evaluations, educate consumers and are able to navigate the State's complicated purchasing system.

As this happened, and contacts were made with consumers, it became very obvious that a huge barrier was the lack of funding. Soon, the centers for independent living, together with the project, went to the State legislature and began advocating for a pot of money to purchase equipment for people when other dollars were not available if they did not qualify for Medicaid or if it was disallowed under private insurance. I am proud to say that today, this pot of money has grown to approximately $800,000 annually that can be spent specifically on devices.

Sustainability was also achieved when the State legislature appropriated State funding to continue the access coordinators. Now, even if the Tech Act were to go away and not be able to coordinate these efforts, the funding comes through the State legislature in a base building block that comes every year. Once that happened, the funding that the State tech project was putting into independent living was able to move on and work with another barrier that the Consumer Council had identified. So that in a way, it was like seed money that helped it get up and going and saw it through so that it was sustainable. This method has been used several times in Utah.

Briefly, in another situation, the project worked with senior centers to provide access to AT devices. Many of the devices they needed were low-tech and readily available, but most often these people were not seeking help from disability-related organizations. They wanted to just go to the place they were already using, which was the senior center. So the obvious answer was the build the capacity of the senior center to meet their needs.

In closing, I just want to tell you that even though the National Council of Independent Living has been critical of some of the practices of tech projects, the governing board has concluded that there is a definite need for continued Federal legislation to make assistive technology devices and services more accessible.

There are several points that we believe must be in place for this to work. The project must view itself as a coordinating entity, not build itself up as the provider of technology and the provider of evaluation services but as the coordinating entity to build capacity in existing programs.

The legislation must maintain a systems change component, and each initiative to build the system should be placed within an existing, ongoing program.

As changes are implemented, resources must be developed from sources other than the Tech Act program. this will ensure a permanent solution.

I have attached with my written testimony a summary of the steps that I have discussed about the Utah project and also the NCIL position paper on the Tech Act.

I would like to thank you for this opportunity that you have provided me today, and I would welcome any questions that you may have.

The CHAIRMAN. Well, thank you for very excellent testimony, and I will come back to you.

[The prepared statement of Ms. Rowley follows:]

PREPARED STATEMENT OF COREY L. ROWLEY

Senator Jeffords, members of the Senate Committee on Labor and Human Resources, and friends, I appreciate the invitation to testify on the need for new assistive technology legislation. As chairperson of the National Council on Independent Living Assistive Technology Task Force, I have worked with people from around the country on issues related to assistive technology. As a Systems Advocacy Coordinator for an Independent Living Center, I have been active in the state of Utah on efforts related to assistive technology. I have had an opportunity to work with people with disabilities, advocates, agencies, service providers and legislators to improve the assistive technology system in Utah. As a consumer, who has used assistive technology for a non-visible disability, I have had first-hand experience with the value and need for assistive technology devices.

I became involved in the national discussion about technology legislation when I approached the governing board of the National Council on Independent Living (NCIL) about the Tech Act. I was very surprised at their reaction. Although assistive technology is a critical issue for centers for independent living (CIL's), many centers were not working with their State tech projects. Members of the board were critical of the way things were happening in their states, even though the systems change focus of the Tech Act and the advocacy role of Independent Living created a natural partnership. This surprised me, because I have been closely involved in the efforts of the Utah Assistive Technology Program, and we were anxious to see these efforts continue.

The Utah Assistive Technology Program (UATP) funded by the Tech Act has been in existence for nine years. It has reached a point in our State that we are able to look back and evaluate some of the steps that we have taken to create permanent systems change in Utah's assistive technology system.

- The first factor that proved to be critical was that the project was not placed within a state agency. The Tech Act called for changes to be made in education, Medicaid and Vocational Rehabilitation assistive technology policies. The effectiveness of the project and the ability to make those changes is compromised when you work within that system. In Utah's case, the tech project is in a University Affiliated Program which is independent of the state service system.
- Representation from each state agency that provided services to people with disabilities is required on the Management and Implementation (M & I) Board. In almost every situation, members are the directors of those agencies, not substitutes

without decision-making authority. When the M&I board discusses a better way to get coverage for equipment from Medicaid, the Medicaid director is there to respond. The Utah Assistive Technology Program staff are staff to the Board, not to a service agency.

A Utah Assistive Technology Program Consumer Council was established. All Consumer Council members are people with disabilities or parent advocates. The consumers meet and identify the barriers surrounding Assistive technology in Utah. They report these issues to the M&I Board. The Board is required to respond in writing on activities undertaken in response to Consumer Council recommendations. The Consumer Council meets as an individual council and also as members of the M&I Board with equal voting rights. I should also point out that the bylaws of the M&I Board state that the Consumer Council has veto rights over any action of the Board.

• One of the most important elements of the Utah Project is that each initiative is required to be sustainable. This was done to ensure that as progress is made, it would continue, even if the Tech Act were to sunset. As each barrier was identified and worked on, the project kept in mind that it was a time-limited project. Not only did the project need to address the barrier, but plan how the solution would continue after UATP was gone. As a result, UATP sustainability activities focused on state funding, policy changes, and state legislative changes. Tech Act dollars were spent on each initiative with the clear understanding that when continuing support was found, the UATP funds would cease. It is important to note that the responsibility for sustainability remained with UATP and was not passed on to the subcontractors.

In many instances around the country, a Tech Act project gives a contract to an assistive technology service entity with the expectation that when the contract ends, the entity will be able to sustain the change or maintain the program. While this may sound good, it has rarely worked out. Often, the entity does not have the capacity to find other resources to support it. Even though the subcontractor can be part of the answer, the responsibility to provide resources and coordination should be left with the Tech Act project.

• Hand in hand with sustainability are efforts to build capacity within existing programs. To build capacity, you have to utilize an ongoing community resource and enhance its capability to address assistive technology issues. As you change a program's AT capabilities, you integrate technology into the services that are already being provided. Now the person needing either a piece of equipment or an assistive technology service can go to an existing community service agency and obtain a variety of services, including assistive technology services.

In Utah, this happens in our centers for independent living. The Tech Act project and the Utah Office of Rehabilitation developed a system of Assistive Technology Coordinators. Each Coordinator conducts evaluations, educates consumers and navigates the state's complicated purchasing system. Contacts with consumers on assistive technology issues have emphasized the need to find funding to purchase devices when people were not eligible for other programs. Soon a legislative request was made for state dollars to buy assistive technology for consumers of independent living. That pot of state money has increased over the years and is now approximately $800,000 annually.

Sustainability was achieved when the state legislature appropriated state funding to continue the Assistive Technology Coordinators. Now the AT Coordinators are completely funded by the state of Utah. It is important to remember that while centers for independent living were involved and part of this long-term solution, the responsibility to secure ongoing support stayed with UATP. After funding was acquired the dollars that initiated the Independent Living AT Coordinator program were available to address other barriers identified by consumers. This method has been used several times in Utah.

• In another situation, the project worked with senior citizen centers to provide access to assistive devices and provide AT information for people who are older. Many of the devices they needed were low-tech and readily available. Most often, these people were not seeking help from disability-related organizations and it became obvious that the solution was to help the senior centers address this need.

States must realize that building up the tech project to be the answer to all assistive technology needs is not an effective long-term solution. Utah planned and carried out activities with a clear understanding that we were responsible to create system and policy changes that would be in place beyond the tech project itself. As you can see, the Tech Act has the capacity to bring additional funding, create and enhance policies, and empower people with disabilities. The need to continue a coordinated effort is clear.

The world of assistive technology is rapidly changing. As new communication devices, wheelchairs, transportation, communications technology and others are developed, people with disabilities need access to these resources. Equally as important as the devices themselves are the policy changes that are taking place. Assistive technology is quickly becoming integrated into existing legislation, as it should be. Managed care has changed the way people access devices through their private insurance. These and other changes make a statewide, coordinated effort critical. Only as people at the local level hold programs responsible will our laws be implemented as they were truly intended.

Even though the National Council on Independent Living has been critical of some of the practices of the tech projects, the governing board has concluded that there is a definite need for continued federal assistance to make assistive technology devices and services more accessible. It is NCIL's belief that technology-related legislation is vital and that NCIL needs to be a part of the efforts to improve legislation that will hold states accountable for outcomes.

We believes that in order to have legislation that will be successful in all states, this congress must consider technology-related legislation which includes the following points:

• The project must view itself as a coordinating entity rather than a service provider.

• The legislation must maintain a systems change component.

• Each initiative to build the assistive technology system capacity should be placed within an existing, ongoing service program.

• As changes are implemented, resources must be developed from sources other than the Tech Act program. This will ensure a permanent solution.

Strong federal technology-related legislation, coordination at the state level, and decisions being made locally by the people who need the services can create an assistive technology system second to none. I would like to thank you for the opportunity you have provided for me to emphasize the need for assistive technology legislation and would welcome any questions that you may have.

SUMMARY

Factors that Have Contributed to the Success of the Utah Assistive Technology Program

• Utah focused on three basic principles:

1. Statewide systems change by pursuing state appropriations and legislation to ensure sustainability.

2. Efforts were focused on building capacity in existing programs that were ongoing and established as a resource within their communities.

3. The focus of the Tech Act was used to pursue additional funding from federal and state sources. For example, a federal grant was received to develop inservice training on AT. In another situation, a federal supplemental appropriation was received to develop a system that would expand rural access to AT.

• The Tech Act Program was not placed in a state agency.

• Representation from each state agency that provided services to people with disabilities was required as a member of the Management and Implementation (M&I) Board. Tech Project employees are staff to this Board.

• A Consumer Council was established. Members identified barriers related to assistive technology and made reports to the M&I Board. The consumers met as an individual council and also were members of the M&I Board with equal voting rights.

• Financial support was provided in order to develop a system that would alleviate a barrier that had been identified by the Consumer Council. After the capacity to change the problem had been built and ongoing support established, the funds were pulled back and used to start a new initiative.

• All activities were required to be sustainable. This requirement cannot be given to individual grantees. It must be an activity coordinated by the Tech Project.

• Consumer participation and responsiveness has been vital. Coordination with organizations that represent consumers and that are comprised of consumers has been a method in achieving this.

COREY ROWLEY, CHAIR

NATIONAL COUNCIL ON INDEPENDENT LIVING

ASSISTIVE TECHNOLOGY TASK FORCE

1916 Wilson Blvd., Suite 209

ARLINGTON, VA 22201

(703) 525-3406

NCIL@TSBBS02.TNET.COM

THE NATIONAL COUNCIL ON INDEPENDENT LIVING (NCIL)

POSITION ON THE TECHNOLOGY RELATED ASSISTANCE FOR INDIVIDUALS WITH DISABILITIES ACT OF 1988 (TECH ACT)

The National Council on Independent Living (NCIL) is a national membership organization comprised of Centers for Independent Living, persons with disabilities, independent living advocates and organizations supporting the principles of independent living.

NCIL was founded in 1982 for the purpose of advocating for improved national policies affecting all persons with disabilities. These policies include but are not limited to, housing, education, transportation, personal assistance, air travel, communication, architectural accessibility, reform of vocational rehabilitation systems, and social security.

Working from a premise that society, not people with disabilities, needs to be fixed, independent living advocates have demanded that people with disabilities have control over the options and methods which bring them the greatest independence and control over their own lives. This includes greater authority over both administration and services designed to benefit people with disabilities. Centers for Independent Living became the first group of private, non-profit organizations to exemplify this principle, known as consumer control.

NCIL believes that there are certain basic values which must be incorporated into any system that promotes integration of persons with disabilities into the mainstream of society. These values must includes consumer control of programs or services and a cross-disability orientation which assures that persons with all types of disabilities receive equitable services.

NCIL's support is contingent upon the inclusion of the independent living values in the Tech Act or in any proposed legislation that continues to address assistive technology.

HISTORY OF THE TECH ACT

People with disabilities rely on assistive technology (AT) everyday. It is an integral part of many peoples lives. The Tech Act and the changes it can promote are central to the system of supports that people with disabilities need. Many Centers for Independent Living (CIL's) have not been satisfied with the methods and outcomes that tech Act projects have used in developing AT services and policies to meet the needs of consumers. Some projects have turned into service providers themselves. Although this may have helped some people, it did nothing to create a long term solution. Others chose to contract away the responsibility. There are some states that have been successful and others that have made progress in specific areas. NCIL believes that responsible technology related legislation is necessary and can be developed using experiences from the past. The goal of technology related legislation must be to assist each state in creating a consumer controlled AT system, not to perpetuate individual projects.

When the Act first became law in 1988 it was intended to sunset after five years. As that time approached it became obvious that the world of assistive technology (AT) was developing rapidly and constantly changing. In 1994 the Tech Act was reauthorized for an additional 5 years with a new direction. The amendments of 1994 required states to emphasize activities that were likely to produce permanent systems change in the area of assistive technology. The new direction from the amendments, together with the original intent of the law to involve consumers with all disabilities and background in every aspect of developing AT policy created the possibility for a natural partnership among CILs, SILCs and individual state tech projects.

Many CILs have developed expertise in the area of assistive technology. One of the four core services for Independent Living is systems advocacy. Center's have a direct connection to consumers that are affected by assistive technology programs and services. These issues make CILs an obvious ally in producing permanent and positive systems change.

The 1994 reauthorization called for funding to be reduced in year nine and ten and then discontinue. This was implemented with the assumption that at the end of year ten, states would have made significant progress in the area of assistive technology that would be in effect when the state project phased out. The first eight states that were funded are now in their ninth year. States were awarded grants based on an RFP process. They were given out over a number of years. Therefore, states are in different years of funding cycles. With the act slated to sunset in 1999, NCIL believes that it is necessary to implement a two-pronged approach to address the future of the Tech Act.

FUTURE OF THE TECH ACT

Should all states receive ten years of funding?

Because current provisions in the Tech Act call for it to sunset in 1999, not all states would have funding to complete a full ten years of project.

NCIL supports ten years for all states providing that the reauthorized legislation requires all state projects to work with Centers for Independent Living in a substantive way (collaboration/contracts for advocacy, consumers and/or staff members of CILs on governing boards of projects, etc.). The legislation must define substantive and set reporting requirements.

Is there adequate reason to request another cycle of funding or alternative assistive technology legislation beyond ten years?

NCIL believes that each state must have a coordinating entity dedicated to the issues of assistive technology for the following reasons:

- The dynamic nature of assistive technology results in constant and rapid change.
- Advocacy needs to be done to ensure assistive technology is addressed in each area and becomes integrated into existing laws so that the barriers related to assistive technology begin to disappear.
- As laws such as Individuals with Disabilities Education Act, Rehabilitation Act, Older American Act and others begin to address assistive technology issues, advocacy will need to be done to ensure that the intent of the laws are carried out. This will only happen as individual states advocate with their own local school districts, vocational rehabilitation agencies, medicaid administrators and others.
- Constant changes in the medical arena need to be addressed. When the Tech Act was first enacted managed care was only on the horizon. Managed care, as it relates to assistive technology, demands efforts to increase assistive technology access.
- The future of assistive technology is unknown. An entity with the charge of addressing issues proactively could avoid future barriers.

NCIL believes there is a need for specific technology related legislation to continue beyond 1999. With regard to the original sunset intent of the Tech Act, NCIL believes that could still be honored as long as legislation is developed that would support system change activities in each state.The focus must remain on systems advocacy that results in a permanent assistive technology system in each state which meets the needs of people with disabilities.

NCIL makes the following recommendations for technology related legislation. These requirements will ensure that support will be given to a community based group with a focus on building a network of advocates to develop a consumer directed AT system in each state.

The process for determining a coordinating entity to support the activities of the legislation must meet the following criteria:

- governing council comprised of 51 percent persons with disabilities
- substantive collaboration with specific organizations such as centers for independent living, protection and advocacy programs, senior citizens centers, statewide independent living councils, university affiliated programs, developmental disability councils, rehabilitation advisory councils, advocacy groups and others actively involved in assistive technology
- a focus that is cross-disability and cross-cultural in nature

Future legislation must ensure that all states:

1. Demonstrate they are building capacity in existing programs

NCIL believes this is the component that can make future legislation (whether it is to continue the current tech act or develop something new) successful. The project should view itself as a coordinating entity with the responsibility to work with existing programs to integrate assistive technology options into ongoing opportunities. This would ensure permanent systems change. There is no need to duplicate efforts within the program itself. Existing programs, such as Centers for Independent Living, Senior Citizen Centers and others have developed a role in the community and will be in existence to continue the ongoing assistive technology activities that are developed.

2. Continue focus of the Tech Act to ensure that as services are developed within existing programs there is a requirement to make them self supporting.

This will ensure that new opportunities are permanent and result in a state that is equipped to meet the assistive technology needs of people with disabilities. Although difficult, this will ensure that as the legislation sunsets or changes the gains that have been made will be ongoing and not lost.

3. Develop data collection and evaluation methods that reflect the intended outcome of the project.

This will ensure progress and accountability. The data must be monitored and reviewed by peers regularly. All states must meet specific criteria in order to receive continued funding. Standards and indicators should be developed.

4. Develop a loan program (often called a foundation) for people with disabilities to borrow money with low interest and low payments for the purchase of assistive technology.

Although some states have done this, many have not. This helps people that do not qualify for purchasing assistance by guaranteeing a loan that is more easily repaid. This also helps people who do not qualify for assistance from other sources.

The CHAIRMAN. Mr. Gashel, it is good to see you again. Please proceed.

Mr. GASHEL. Thank you, Senator Jeffords, and also, thank you for the reminder that on issues like this, our association goes back many years—in fact, prior to the Tech Act.

The CHAIRMAN. Yes, that is right.

Mr. GASHEL. It is a real pleasure for me to be here today to talk about some of the programs of the National Federation of the Blind. Let me just say that in my written statement, I express the frightening possibility that developments in information technology and in the Information Age could be more profoundly disabling for blind people than perhaps anything that we have experienced heretofore, and I want to begin by explaining that just a little bit.

It occurs to me to make that statement because when you realize that the current trend in visual displays and point-and-click technology is really the direction in which information technology has gone.

The example I give in my written statement is the simple operation of a television set, which I used to be able to do pretty well; you cannot do it anymore if you cannot see every element of that television set, because more and more of the functions are going over to onscreen menus, as you may have realized. So, not only did it used to be difficult to operate a VCR, but it is now getting hard just to operate a simple television set. It ought not be this way, and as long as we have onscreen menus as the only way to manipulate the system, it will be this way.

This telephone that I have with me is a cellular telephone. This is a digital telephone, and I can operate it for the most part because it has push-buttons on it, but let me tell you, once I get this telephone turned on and try to operate it, most of the choices I have to make appear on an onscreen menu. Now, most of the time, I can actually make a call on this telephone, but it takes me one or two tries, and a lot of times, I get the operator, who says you cannot make an international call on this telephone—and I do not want to make an international call; I am just trying to call Baltimore. But the problem is that if I cannot see the onscreen menu, I am attempting to make an international call when I do not even want to make an international call.

This telephone could just as well have been devised, since it is entirely digital, with a speaker right out of it which would say to me what this menu says right here. But the manufacturer did not think to do it. It was not a priority, and it needs to be a priority.

The examples of this kind of thing are so pervasive in our lives that I see blind people every day who are losing their jobs when they were trained to work in information technology. It is enough that blind people have now begun to say, "There ought to be a law," and by George, there ought to be a law, and it ought to be an access law. That is what the Tech Act ought to look to in the future.

Now I want to briefly tell you a little bit about some of the initiatives of the National Federation of the Blind in terms of access, because we believe there are certain things that we in the private sector can do without a law to demonstrate the possible and the positive.

For one thing, we have set up a consumer evaluation center. Now, certainly, this type of thing is perhaps contemplated under the Technology Assistance Act, but it is not going on very much. We have set up a consumer evaluation center and also a model technology development effort as well. We use these efforts to promote nonvisual access. So for example, in the evaluation center, we buy—we do not have it given to us—we buy and test software and devices which provide nonvisual access, including Braille output and speech output, in using computers.

Our commitment is to buy one of everything and to test it in a nonmarketing, absolutely consumer-controlled context. Therefore, manufacturers who develop nonvisual access technology——

The CHAIRMAN. Excuse me, Jim. I am going to have to interrupt you to go and vote. I will be back as fast as I can.

The committee will stand in recess.

[Recess.]

The CHAIRMAN. Sorry to interrupt you, Jim. Please proceed.

Mr. GASHEL. Thanks a lot.

As I was saying, in the evaluation center, we buy one of every software or hardware device and test it in a nonmarketing, absolutely consumer-controlled context. Therefore, every manufacturer of nonvisual access technology is on notice—or, for that matter, of visual access technology, including our friends at Microsoft—is absolutely on notice that we will be testing the devices and the software that they make, and we will be publishing consumer reports on many of the items. With that capacity, our own consumer evaluation center, blind people are taking charge of shaping the technology which will meet our needs today and in the future.

This type of capacity-building to ensure consumers an independent voice in testing and speaking out on the technology that works for us ought to be a part of both the technology assistance programs and the Act that makes them possible.

Speaking of capacity-building, Mr. Chairman, there ought to also be support for consumer models in technology development. The NFB's services called Newsline and Jobline illustrate that consumers can also take an active part in technology development, and my written statement has details on these services, so I will just briefly summarize.

Newsline is access to newspapers, and it is really spoken word access to newspapers. We present a spoken word edition of many national papers and lots of local newspapers on the telephone. So that with Newsline, callers in 38 local dialing areas—and I cite many of them in my written statement—and soon to be 42 areas can have their newspapers immediately available on the telephone, all by way of computer and without human intervention, and they can have it 24 hours a day, 7 days a week. I do not know about your newspaper, but my paper never ends up in the rose bushes or in the mud; it is always on the telephone. I can read what I choose and when I choose to read it just by pressing the keys on the telephone.

This shows the possibility of nonvisual access technology and the great potential of where we are. Unfortunately, not enough of this sort of thing is done.

Let me say that thanks to efforts by the technology assistance program in Maryland, we have also been able to develop a special use channel that goes along with Newsline to present local information, and I would say that our technology assistance program in Maryland is really committed to the principles of nonvisual access and has helped to make it happen in our State, and this is contributing to the entire national effort as well.

Our newest service, which is Jobline, is really exciting. It is an extension of the Newsline technology. With Jobline, it is possible to search a national database of 70,000 job announcements. Again, this is done just by using the touch-tone telephone, and the job announcements which meet the caller's qualifications are spoken to the caller on the telephone. The match is determined by a personal profile which the caller inputs for himself, and the job announcements come from America's Job Bank on the internet; that is something you can see using such facilities as Internet Explorer, but if you are blind, now with Jobline, you can hear it on the telephone.

We have also received great cooperation from the U.S. Department of Labor in making the Jobline service possible. With an appropriation that was included in the Department of Labor's budget for the current fiscal year, we are anticipating the actual implementation of Jobline in 40 States during the next 12 to 18 months.

Incidentally, since job orders are not copyrighted text, they are not subject to the same copyright restrictions as news articles would be on Newsline, where we have to provide that service only to blind people when we work with the newspapers on that. But in job orders, this is something that can be made available to everyone.

This brings me to my concluding point, Mr. Chairman, which has to do with the potential for nonvisual access and universal design in the future. Our experience in developing products such as Newsline and Jobline shows that access need not be and should not be conditioned on a person's ability to see. Accepting that view and following through on it is really a matter of commitment and priority. Lip service in a way that treats access as an afterthought—which is, frankly, what has happened in a lot of cases—is just not good enough, and it is not acceptable, and it ought not be acceptable to the entities of Government which buy a lot of this technology and spend hundreds of millions of dollars doing so.

Jobline resulted from a commitment by the U.S. Secretary of Labor, Secretary Reich, when he said that the one-stop service delivery system in work force development would follow access principles and be fully accessible to persons with disabilities. This says to me that the commitment must come not just from the manufacturers, but ultimately from the major league buyers and users of information technology as well. This must include leadership by entities of Government, as I said, to underscore and enforce the principles of nonvisual access and universal design.

Providing the impetus for this leadership ought to be the mission of the technology assistance program, Mr. Chairman. And by the way, I think the Department of Education and NIDRR are doing an excellent job of administering the current law that they have to administer, but in the future, they have got to have much greater authority in the area of promoting nonvisual access and universal design, and I hope the amendments will lead in that direction.

Thank you very much.

[The prepared statement of Mr. Gashel follows:]

PREPARED STATEMENT OF JAMES GASHEL

Mr. Chairman, my name is James Gashel. I am appearing in this hearing today on behalf of the National Federation of the Blind. My address is 1800 Johnson Street, Baltimore, Maryland 21230.

I want to begin by thanking you for the opportunity to testify on reauthorization of the Technology-Related Assistance for Individuals With Disabilities Act because concerns regarding technology have become crucial for blind people. Before I explain that statement in greater depth, I think it would be helpful for you to have some relevant background information on the National Federation of the Blind. First and foremost, the Federation is a membership organization of blind people. All of our leaders and the vast majority of our members are blind. Therefore, we are often referred to as the "voice of the nation's blind."

In the terms in which the Tech Act identifies the various interests, the National Federation of the Blind represents the organized consumer of assistance and services. "Organized" is one of the key words in our vocabulary, because the Federation consists of state affiliates representing every state, the District of Columbia, and Puerto Rico. We also have local chapters in most sizable population areas in the United States. Then in addition to this, we also have several special interest divisions which blind people join to address particular concerns and needs. Overall, our total membership is more than 50,000 strong nationally.

Turning to technology, which is the subject of this hearing, as far as blind people are concerned, the issue is "access." In fact, I think there would be wide agreement that this is perhaps the most compelling and challenging issue of the times for us. In speaking of access, I am referring to the capacity to receive, use, and send information. Since we live in an age in which information and the ability to compete for jobs and opportunities have become interrelated, it should be obvious why access has become a matter of compelling concern for blind people, but there is more to the issue than that alone.

The pessimist would tell you that the world of video screens and graphical presentations is exploding around us to the extent that if you can't see it, you can't use it. But, from the point of view of the optimist, the possibility of access through alternative nonvisual technologies is a reasonable and realistic expectation. This is why the National Federation of the Blind takes the optimistic view, although the fears of the pessimist have plenty of support.

Mr. Chairman, I realize that access in using information technology is not necessarily the focus of the present law. However, the need for statutory provisions on access (and particularly on nonvisual access) could not be more compelling. I say this because of the growing extent to which the effective use of information technology is a controlling factor in our ability to communicate.

Speaking to this situation as a blind person, I can tell you that the prospect of being locked out technologically from professional, commercial, and social interaction is a frightening and very real possibility. I confronted the fact that this could happen quite recently when I checked into a hotel, got to my room, and found that I was completely unable to operate the television set. The reason was that just moving from channel to channel was not possible without being able to see and read the on-screen menu. So, at least on that occasion, I couldn't even listen to C-Span.

In the latter part of the 1960's when I was preparing to go to work, a great many of my blind friends and colleagues were encouraged to pursue employment opportunities in computer technology. This occurred to such an extent that computer programming was actually becoming a modern-day stereotyped occupational placement for the blind.

But now, in an environment in which nonvisual access may be impossible or difficult at best to achieve, the same people who have worked successfully on a par with their sighted peers for many years have become technological casualties. Also, the prospects for young blind people to pursue careers in systems development and programming are surprisingly more limited, even though many employers complain about a need for trained personnel in this area.

I point this out to illustrate how access has become the crucial issue of the age. Just sit down at any computer or walk up to a public information kiosk, close your eyes, and try to use it. Then, think about the fact that devices such as these are rapidly becoming the centerpiece of information exchange.

Since the situation as I have described it is unquestionably becoming a fact of everyday life, the barriers to full participation of blind people in the society of the future must be faced today. In the view of the National Federation of the Blind, that challenge—the challenge of leading our society toward universal access in information technology—ought to be part of the reauthorized legislation.

With this as a foundation, Mr. Chairman, I would now like to describe two important contributions which consumer-led initiatives can make toward achieving the goal of universal access, including nonvisual access. The first of these is consumer-led evaluation of technology, and the second is consumer-led development of technology. When I use the term "consumer," I am referring in our case to leadership provided by blind people who are in positions of accountability to blind people. This is something which is fundamental to the National Federation of the Blind, because blind people are the members and leaders of our organization at all levels.

Evaluation of technology in a setting which is entirely controlled by blind consumers is something which we value as a top priority for our movement. This is why we established the International Braille and Technology Center for the Blind and have continued to support the Center through its growth since it opened in November, 1990.

The present facility occupies 20,000 square feet and includes two hundred separate work stations. The equipment and software which is installed and operational includes Braille embossers; computers with synthesized speech; Braille and speech-output notetakers; stand-alone reading machines; computer-based text-to-speech reading systems; computers with access to the Internet; and a variety of other single-purpose devices to meet particular needs.

Our operating protocol in maintaining the Center is to buy at least one of every Braille and speech-output device or system which is sold for the specialized purpose of nonvisual access. The challenging word is "buy"—not "accept" or "receive"—but "buy." And the commitment we have made is to continue to buy the devices and relevant software which are being introduced to the market as access technology for blind people each and every year.

Our investment in technology to date is about $2 million and climbing. We find the money to support this effort because we want to be completely independent from manufacturers or marketing interests. This is essential if the advice we give or reports we publish are to be regarded as credible. Also, the evaluation work which occurs day-in and day-out at the Center is entirely in the hands of blind people. This is true of our members who volunteer their time and talents to this effort and the staff who devote their full time and attention to support the effort.

As a result, anyone who may want to know about the device or software best suited to meet a particular individualized need can contact the Center to obtain the information or visit the Center for a personal inspection and on-site comparison of features. Inquiries by telephone, mail, and the Internet are handled in a growing volume every day. Personal inspection tours by visitors from everywhere in the U.S. and many foreign countries occur in a steady stream as well.

If I had to pick just one important contribution that has been made by this facility, I would point to the comprehensive presentation of access devices and software in a non-marketing context, where consumers—not inventors—are the experts.

While such activities are possibly envisioned under the present authority of the Tech Act, I would say that greater emphasis should be placed on support for model consumer-led evaluation programs such as this.

But consumer-led evaluation, without moving to the next step of consumer-led development, may not be sufficient. At least this is our experience. So, the National Federation of the Blind has decided to lead by example in the creation of technology as well as in its evaluation.

Several examples of this come to mind, but our service known as Newsline(r) and another application of the same technology known as Jobline(r) are perhaps the most prominent current initiatives now underway. I will describe this technology briefly and be happy to show it to you during the exposition being held this afternoon. Once again, the leadership provided by blind consumers has made this technology possible.

Remember what I said about "access." That's what Newsline(r) and Jobline(r) are all about. Newsline(r) means access to newspapers. We created that service to place blind people on an equal footing with others in access to the print media, and we are now working hard to get communities of every size throughout the nation connected to the service.

This, in fact, is happening because Newsline(r) uses the standard touch-tone telephone as the means of distribution. So, we are hard at work in the effort to establish local dial-in sites in every state and as many local dialing areas as possible. At present there are 38 (and soon to be 42) Newsline(r) centers.

Areas currently served include New York; Los Angeles; Chicago and most of Illinois; the District of Columbia; Maryland and Northern Virginia; Columbus, Ohio; the major cities in Iowa; Dallas, Houston (and other parts of Texas); Salt Lake City, Utah; Chattanooga, Tennessee; Boise, Idaho; Minneapolis, Minnesota; and many more. States in which the service will soon be added include Connecticut, Wisconsin and West Virginia.

The papers carried on Newsline* include USA TODAY, the Washington Post, the Los Angeles Times, the New York Times, the Chicago Tribune, the Toronto Globe and Mail, and several other papers which are distributed in local areas only. The technology which makes Newsline(r) possible involves receiving news text from cooperating media partners over the Internet, converting the text for presentation in a synthetic speech format, and distribution of the converted text files to the appropriate local access points.

When the process is working as it should—which it does most of the time—everything occurs automatically. Therefore, when I sit down to read the morning paper in Baltimore, I am able to choose from most of the papers listed, and the editions just reaching the newsstands for that day are immediately available to me at the touch of a button. Moreover, I can read the sports page, the editorials, the national news, or whatever I choose, when I choose.

In fact, as Newsline(r) has developed and grown, we have probably outdone ourselves in demonstrating the great potential of nonvisual and universal access. How many of you have your local paper plus five or six national papers all at your finger tips each day at 6:00 a.m? Besides, the editions that I receive never end up in the rose bushes or the mud!

Before I talk briefly about Jobline(r), I should mention that Newsline(r) has benefited from support provided through the Tech Act. This has been true in Maryland where the state Technology Assistance Program helped us with funds to develop a method for a local-content channel to supplement the newspapers.

This support and the encouragement we have received in working with personnel from the Maryland Technology Assistance Program provide a model relationship for the advancement of nonvisual access. To their credit, the program officials in Maryland have been outstanding in their outreach on behalf of our consumer-led access initiatives. Partnerships such as this speak to the potential of the Tech Act and should be replicated throughout the country.

This brings me to the most recent version of the Newsline(r)-type technology, which is Jobline(r). Again, the concept is universal (and particularly nonvisual) access, and the content of the service is not news text but job orders. The data base which is used is input from the public job service, known on the Internet as America's Job Bank.

With Jobline(r), America's Job Bank can talk to anyone on a standard touch-tone telephone. We solved the problem of searching a national data base of 70,000 jobs by means of a personal profile which each caller sets up independently in using the service. Then, at literally the touch of a button, the system selects and presents only those job announcements which match the job-seeking caller's profile. Its truly a wonderful system, and I hope you will come and see or listen to it this afternoon.

48-228 98 - 3

As for implementation, this service would not be possible without cooperation from the U.S. Department of Labor. I realize that this cooperation should be expected, but I want you to be aware of it all the same. And speaking of cooperation, the Congress, too, has played a part in this development by setting aside $3 million from the amount appropriated for labor market information for the current fiscal year.

As a result, we can now anticipate that this service will become available statewide in as many as forty states within the next several months. Once again, I should say that Maryland has been the first to install it. This shows that a commitment to nonvisual access is becoming a source of pride in that state, and the Technology Assistance Program is working with us to make it that way.

Mr. Chairman, you have asked me to comment on factors which impede the use of universal access principles in the design of new technology. This would be a good question for a company of the size and influence of Microsoft, but here is what I would say. It all comes down to commitment and priority.

Take for example the creation of a public service such as America's Job Bank on the Internet. According to one person who was candid enough to say it this way, disability (not to mention blindness) did not even make their radar screen. That was the case until Secretary Reich appeared before an audience at Gallaudet University in October, 1996, and committed his Department to a one-stop service delivery system that is fully accessible to all with state-of-the-art technology. Jobline* is at least one result of that commitment.

Could the presentation of information in electronic forms be generally accessible to persons who cannot see? With the experience we have had in creating products such as Newsline(r) and Jobline(r), my answer would be not just "yes," but emphatically "yes." In my opinion this will not be done, however, until the prominent leaders in technology today make the commitment such as Secretary Reich did. Then, having made the commitment, they must back it up with the resources needed so that universal access becomes a corporate priority.

The challenge of getting to that point is substantial but not beyond our reach. The challenge is substantial because developments in technology are largely being driven by the goal of beating the competition to the market. Therefore, since most consumers can see and respond to visual cues, visual display technology has top priority in product design. Alternative access for nonvisual use may be considered at some point, but usually (if ever) as an afterthought.

This will continue to be the case until the leaders in technology development are compelled to include nonvisual access features in the design of new products from the beginning. I use the term "compelled" advisedly, because designing alternative access features competes with the need to sell and invent more products. That's what technology companies are all about.

If it would ever be possible to concentrate the total resources which blind people can bring to the table in buying information technology, the combined purchasing power would be insignificant to a company of the size of Microsoft or other major leaders. However, the combined strength of governmental entities is not insignificant in this market.

Also, it is reasonable to expect governmental entities to insist upon having nonvisual and other universal design features included in the information technology which they buy. This is reasonable because of the use of public funds. Therefore, laws, such as the proposed revisions to section 508 of the Rehabilitation Act must be passed, although the loopholes should be closed and the language should be stronger.

States, too, should commit themselves to procurement of information technology which must include nonvisual and other universal access features in the design. Acceptance of funds under the Tech Act should also mean that the state will join the effort to put such procurement requirements in place.

Returning to my statement about the observable trend in information technology, the consequences of failing to plan for universal design are really quite frightening. Just consider the challenge still being met in our society to overcome barriers to persons with disabilities that were caused in the design of the physical environment. Dealing with situations such as this is always far more expensive and often less effective than anticipating the problem and solving it before the fact.

In the case of our evolving technology, Mr. Chairman, the chance to plan for universal use still exists, and there is hope. That hope will die, however, unless there is a genuine national commitment to access which is backed by government and joined by the industry and consumers. Creating the leadership needed to support and fulfill this commitment must be a goal which the technology assistance program both expresses and embraces.

In fact, I would say that the expression and enforcement of a commitment to access ought to be the central purpose of the amendments presented and passed this year.

On behalf of the National Federation of the Blind, I thank you.

The CHAIRMAN. Thank you for your usual very powerful and explicit statement. I appreciate it very much.

Ms. Rowley, if we were to authorize Federal funding for limited core activities for tech projects that have exceeded 10 years of Federal funding, which core activities would be most important?

Ms. ROWLEY. I believe that the consumers in our State, as they met as a Consumer Council, came to the conclusion that holding service entities accountable for what they are supposed to do as part of their laws, such as Medicaid, vocational rehabilitation and all of those, is one of them.

Another one is that they continue to say that lack of funding for equipment is a barrier. Whether that means creating private partnerships with local communities or with your State legislature or however it needs to happen in each State—I would be remiss to think that all States could go to the State legislature and get the funding; however, we have an extremely conservative legislature that has taken on assistive technology as something that they see a huge need for and have been extremely supportive of in a nonpartisan way. So funding, holding current entities responsible, and capacity-building in a place where consumers are already going.

I think that as long as we continue to see assistive technology on one side and other services on another, we will never get a good mix. But if someone can go and apply for services for independent living and at the same time have their assistive technology needs met, you have created a lot of bang for your buck, and you have helped that consumer get what he or she needed in one area.

The CHAIRMAN. Thank you. That is very helpful.

Mr. Gashel, we are exploring the concept of regional technical assistance centers for assistive technology. The focus of such centers would be to foster interstate collaborations in the area of assistive technology. Would you give us some suggestions about how such centers may be undertaken?

Mr. GASHEL. I think that that is probably a pretty good idea. I would simply say that there ought to be a very strong consumer governance of such centers if that would be possible, and I expect it would be possible if you wrote the law that way. It has certainly been possible in the areas of independent living. But our experience in developing the International Braille and Technology Center for the Blind really proves that consumers ought to take the leadership in evaluation, because after all, we are going to be using the technology, and we do not want these to be medical centers or centers necessarily that are solely operated and controlled by engineers or technology developers. The consumer needs to have the ultimate leadership in this kind of center, and I think they could do a great deal of good if that were the case.

The CHAIRMAN. Thank you.

Time moves on, and we have to move on to another panel. I first want to thank all of you, especially Carol. It was a pleasure meeting you, and I look forward to watching your success. All of you have been very helpful, and I know where to reach Ms. Rowley and

Mr. Gashel, so we will probably be pestering you with a few questions over and beyond today's hearing.

Thank you so much.

Our final panel today includes Lynne Cleveland, who is project director of the Vermont Assistive Technology Project in Waterbury, VT. Next is Cris Fulford, who is the Tech Act Project Manager of the ATTAIN Project in Indianapolis, IN; and Marion Pawlek, who is coordinator of the New Hampshire Assistive Technology Project in Concord, NH

I welcome all of you to the table. Lynne Cleveland comes from my home State of Vermont and is director of the Vermont Assistive Technology Project as well as a co-chair of the National Association of Tech Act Projects. Prior to that, she served two terms in the Vermont House of Representatives. In both of these positions, she has advocated successfully for individuals with disabilities and their families in the Sate of Vermont, and I am delighted that she could be here with us today.

Our second witness will be Cris Fulford, who is director of Assessing Technology Through Awareness in Indiana, ATTAIN, and has directed this $5 million program since 1992. Prior to joining ATTAIN, Cris worked in the field of physical therapy for 6 years. Cris is joined today by her son Craig, a 22-year-old student enrolled in the Business Studies Options Program at Vincennes University. Craig has become a trainer in the ATTAIN Empowerment and Advocacy Program, working with local communities to infuse assistive technology. I am happy that you could join us.

Our final witness is Marion Pawlek, who is currently the project coordinator for the New Hampshire Assistive Technology partnership Program located at the University of New Hampshire's Institute for Disability. She has been with the project since its inception in 1992 and has spearheaded such initiatives as the development of a nonprofit training program, a financial loan program, and a very comprehensive equipment recycling program. We look forward to your testimony.

Shall we start with Ms. Cleveland? It is a pleasure to have you here.

STATEMENTS OF LYNNE CLEVELAND, PROJECT DIRECTOR, VERMONT ASSISTIVE TECHNOLOGY PROJECT, WATERBURY, VT; MARION PAWLEK, PROJECT COORDINATOR, NEW HAMPSHIRE ASSISTIVE TECHNOLOGY PARTNERSHIP PROJECT, CONCORD, NH; AND CRIS FULFORD, TECH ACT PROJECT DIRECTOR, ATTAIN PROJECT, INDIANAPOLIS, IN, ACCOMPANIED BY CRAIG FULFORD, STUDENT AND ATTAIN PROJECT TRAINER

Ms. CLEVELAND. Thank you, Senator Jeffords, and thank you for the yeoman's work that you have done for Vermonters with disabilities through IDEA and the Rehab Act and the Assistive Technology Act, and thank you for the opportunity to speak with you today.

In 1988, when Congress passed the Technology-Related Assistance for Individuals with Disabilities Act, you acknowledged the need for ensuring that individuals with disabilities in all States and Territories would gain knowledge of, access to and funding for assistive technology. Congress recognized that assistive technology is integral to empowering consumers to achieve independence, productivity and inclusion in education, the work force and community life, and that without appropriate assistive technology, the ability of an individual to achieve those goals is severely compromised.

The beauty of the Tech Act is that it is the vehicle through which every State and Territory can respond to the unique needs of consumers in that region yet also share with and learn from 55 other projects with the same primary focus, a focus serving a constituency that is rare among entities meeting the needs of individuals with disabilities in that it serves consumers across age and across disability.

Almost no other program that is in place in every State and Territory has this breadth of focus. Tech Act projects have risen to the challenge not only by forming a collaborative network amongst themselves, but more importantly, by becoming strong collaborative partners with and often subcontractors to State agencies, private businesses, nonprofits such as Centers for Independent Living, United Cerebral Palsy, Easter Seals, university-affiliated programs, and other service providers in their States.

In Vermont, these collaborative partnerships coupled with the Vermont Assistive Technology Project's cross-age and cross-disability focus have yielded dramatic results. Through three regional seating and mobility clinics, we have cut by more than half the amount of time it takes for consumers to receive a wheelchair. In collaboration with Vermont Technical College, we established the Rehabilitation Engineer Technician Program. This is the only program in the Nation that offers a 2-year degree in rehabilitation engineering technology. In 4 short years of this program, here is the discernable difference that the graduates have made in Vermont. One graduate received certification from Medicaid and private insurers to perform repairs on wheelchairs, communication devices and other assistive technology, often at an individual's home. In a rural State like Vermont, this has been a tremendous benefit to housebound persons with disabilities.

Another graduate works with the University-Affiliated Program at the University of Vermont to help schools make appropriate assistive technology choices for their students with multiple and severe disabilities. This has saved schools money by enabling them to make informed choices for students the first time. This particular graduate is funded through a collaborative agreement between the Vermont Tech Act Project and the State Department of Education.

Another graduate works for a private durable medical equipment vendor. Since being hired by this vendor, the vendor reports that consumer satisfaction with the AT purchased through his company has vast improved.

Another graduate works with a nonprofit physical and occupational therapy clinical, helping consumers with computer access. She also serves consumers statewide by working with a demo and tryout laboratory established by the Vermont Tech Act Project.

Vermont is an extremely rural State, with many of its 600,000 citizens located in very small, sometimes very isolated, towns. We have met this service delivery challenge in various ways. Many of the training offered by the AT project and its subcontracts is offered over interactive television at 12 sites spread throughout the State. For consumers, this means a half-an-hour drive to attend training rather than a 3-hour trip.

We also have a web site that offer materials such as our funding guides and loan fund applications, as well as information and referral and local, State and national resources.

We have developed collaborative partnerships with organizations such as the Council of Vermont Elders, the Area Agencies on Aging, and the Center for Independent Living, so that the assistive technology information and access that they do is incorporated into their outreach efforts as well.

Vermont is also developing a nonprofit in order to create an expanded recycling program that involves private vendors of assistive technology and works with Medicaid and private insurance to help consumers get the assistive technology they need while spending dollars wisely. The nonprofit will also be the vehicle through which our information and referral and demo and tryout centers will eventually become self-sustaining without Tech Act dollars.

The Tech Act is ultimately about people. Here are some examples of what the Tech Act has done for Vermonters. For Bill, a man in his mid-thirties who suffered a stroke, assistive technology has enabled him to find gainful employment designing web pages and more important to Bill, assistive technology has enabled him to once more be able to talk with his children and tell them bedtime stories.

For Ray, who lost his vision in mid-life, assistive technology has enabled him to continue at his job as snowplow dispatcher for the State of Vermont.

For Ty, a young teenager born with a visual impairment, assistive technology means that she will be able to pursue her goal of becoming a lawyer.

For Annie, a first-grader with Down's syndrome, assistive technology means that she can access the computer in her regular education classroom and participate in learning games with her peers.

For Lillian, an elder, access to and training on a closed-circuit television, a piece of assistive technology, will enable her to stay in her home instead of having to live in a nursing home.

All of these individuals learned of and received their assistive technology due to Tech Act project activities.

What Congress did not anticipate 10 years ago as the Tech Act was authorized was the impact that the unprecedented rapid developments in the field of mainstream technology would have on the world of assistive technology. New technologies bring new opportunities for consumers with disabilities but also bring new challenges in accessibility and funding. As States try to deal with these challenges, they have relied heavily on the expertise of Tech Act projects to help them develop State policy that meets Federal guidelines while assuring access for all citizens. Again, this is the place where the broad focus of cross-age and cross-disability has made the Tech Act projects an invaluable resource in the respective States.

Many State have recognized the need for continuing the work of Tech Act projects and support their projects through various cash and in-kind contributions, some through State agencies and some through private entities. It is reasonable to expect States to do so. However, without a continuing Federal commitment, there will not be enough resources to continue the work. In areas as fundamental as access to assistive technology, States work best when there is a real partnership at the State and Federal level.

Congress could not have anticipated the seismic shift to managed care and its serious impact on a consumer's access to assistive technology through public and private funding streams. Service delivery systems are not static, and satisfactory resolutions of assistive technology issues that were achieved 5 years ago can be instantaneously changed in the blink of a statute amendment or a policy revision. One court decision can wipe out years of work.

Other continuing challenges include the aging of the general population coupled with an increased expectation of maintaining independence in the home for as long as possible, continuing to build capacity of States to provide quality assistance technology devices and services, and training and developing alternative sources of funding AT as public funding programs decrease or stay level-funded.

The primary challenge for the future is to maintain all the gains made by consumers under the Tech Act while assuring an ongoing ability and expertise to adjust to future developments and changes in the field of assistive technology. The role that Tech Act projects play of collaborative facilitator of best practices is a vital role to maintain, and every State and Territory must have the opportunity to do so. This means a full 10 years' funding under the current Tech Act for every State and Territory as well as some form of assistance to all States and Territories after the full 10 years have transpired.

Our strength is our diversity and the ability of each State to shape a program that meets its unique needs. Our history is rich with experience with all consumers of assistive technology, and we stand ready and able to meet the challenges of the 21st century with increased State responsibility joined with an ongoing national commitment to ensuring that all citizens with disabilities have access to the assistive technology they need to enjoy full and productive lives.

Thank you, Senator Jeffords.

The CHAIRMAN. Thank you very much.

[The prepared statement of Ms. Cleveland follows:]

PREPARED STATEMENT OF LYNNE M. CLEVELAND

In 1988, when Congress passed the "Technology-Related Assistance for Individuals with Disabilities Act" you acknowledged a need for insuring that individuals with disabilities in all states and territories would gain knowledge of, access to, and funding for assistive technology. Congress recognized that AT is integral to empowering consumers to achieve independence, productivity, and inclusion in education, the workforce, and community life and that without appropriate assistive technology the ability of an individual to achieve those goals is severely compromised.

The beauty of the Tech Act is that it is the vehicle through which every state and territory can respond to the unique needs of consumers in that region yet also share with and learn from 55 other projects with the same primary focus—a focus serving a constituency that is rare among entities meeting the needs of individuals with disabilities in that it serves consumers cross-age and cross-disability. Almost no other program that is in place in every state and territory has this breadth of focus. Tech Act Projects have risen to the challenge, not only by forming a collaborative network among themselves but more importantly by becoming strong collaborative partners with (and often subcontractors to) state agencies, private businesses, non-profits such as Centers for Independent Living, United Cerebral Palsy, Easter Seals, University Affiliated Programs, and other service providers in their states.

In Vermont these collaborative partnerships coupled with the Vermont Assistive Technology Project's cross-age and cross-disability focus have yielded dramatic results. Through three regional seating and mobility clinics we have cut by more than half the amount of time it takes for a consumer to receive their wheelchair. In collaboration with Vermont Technical College, we established the Rehabilitation Engineer Technician program. This is the only program in the nation that offers a two-year degree in Rehabilitation Engineering Technology. In four short years here is the discernable difference graduates of this program have made in Vermont:

- One graduate has received certification from Medicaid and private insurers to perform repairs on wheelchairs, communication devices and other assistive technology, at the individuals home. For a rural state this has been a tremendous benefit to housebound persons with disabilities.
- Another graduate works with the UAP program at the University of Vermont to help schools make appropriate AT choices for their students with multiple and severe disabilities. This has saved schools money by enabling them to make informed choices for students the first time. This particular graduate is funded through a collaborative agreement between the VT Tech Act Project and the state Department of Education.
- Another graduate works for a private durable medical equipment vendor. The vendor reports that consumer satisfaction with the AT they purchase has vastly improved.
- Another graduate works with a non-profit physical and occupational therapy clinic, helping consumers with computer access. She also serves consumers statewide by working with a demo and tryout laboratory established by the Tech Act Project.

Vermont is an extremely rural state, with many of its 600,000 citizens located in very small, sometimes isolated towns. We have met this service delivery challenge in various ways. Many of the trainings offered by the AT Project and its subcontractors are offered over interactive TV at twelve sites spread throughout the state. For consumers this means a half-hour drive to attend trainings rather than a three-hour trip. We also have a web-site that offers materials such as our funding guides and loan fund applications, as well as information and referral, and local, state, and national resources. We have developed collaborative partnerships with organizations such as the Council of Vermont Elders, the Area Agencies on Aging and the Center for Independent Living so that assistive technology information and access is incorporated into the outreach that these organizations do.

Vermont is also developing a non-profit in order to create an expanded recycling program that involves private vendors of AT and works with Medicaid and private insurance to help consumers get the AT they need while spending dollars wisely. The non-profit will also be the vehicle through which our information and referral and demo and tryout centers become self-sustaining without Tech Act dollars.

The Tech Act is ultimately about people. Here are some examples of what the Tech Act has done for Vermonters:

- For Bill, a man in his mid-thirties who suffered a stroke, AT has enabled him to find gainful employment designing web pages and, most importantly to Bill; AT has enabled him to once more be able to talk to his children.
- For Ray, who lost his vision in mid-life, assistive technology has enabled him to continue at his job as snowplow dispatcher for the State of Vermont.
- For Ty, a teenager born with a visual impairment, AT means she can pursue her goal of becoming a lawyer.
- For Annie, a first grader with Downs Syndrome, AT means that she can access the computer in her regular education classroom and participate in learning games with her peers.
- For Lillian, an elder, access to and training on a Closed Circuit television (CCTV) will enable to stay in her home instead of having to live in a nursing home.

What Congress did not anticipate ten years ago as the Tech Act was authorized was the impact that the unprecedented rapid developments and changes in the field of mainstream technology would have on the world of assistive technology. New technologies bring new opportunities for consumers with disabilities but also bring new challenges in accessibility and funding. As states try to deal with these challenges they have relied heavily on the expertise of Tech Act projects to help them develop state policy that meets federal guidelines while ensuring access for all citizens. Again this is a place where the broad focus of cross-age and cross-disability has made Tech Act projects an invaluable resource in their respective states. Many states have recognized the need for continuing the work of the Tech Act projects and support projects through various cash and inkind contributions, some through state agencies and some through private entities. It is reasonable to expect states to do so. However, without a continuing federal commitment there will not be enough resources to continue the work. In areas as fundamental as access to assistive technology, states work best when there is a real partnership at the state and federal level.

Congress could not have anticipated the seismic shift to Managed Care and its serious impact on a consumer's access to assistive technology through public and private funding streams. Service delivery systems are not static and satisfactory resolutions of AT issues achieved five years ago can be instantaneously changed in the blink of a statute amendment or policy revision. One court decision can wipe out years worth of work. Other challenges include the aging of the general population coupled with an increased expectation of maintaining independence in the home for as long as possible, continuing to build capacity of states to provide quality assistive technology devices and services, training, and developing alternative sources of funding AT as public funding programs decrease or stay level-funded.

The primary challenge for the future is to maintain all the gains made by consumers under the Tech Act while assuring an ongoing ability and expertise to adjust to future developments and changes in the field of assistive technology. The role that Tech Act projects play of collaborative facilitator of best practices is a vital role to maintain and every state and territory must have the opportunity to do so. This means a full ten years funding under the current Tech Act for every state and territory as well as some form of assistance to all states and territories after the full ten years has transpired. Our strength is our diversity and the ability of each state to shape a program that meets its unique needs. Our history is rich with experience with all consumers of assistive technology and we stand ready and able to meet the challenges of the twenty-first century with increased state responsibility joined with an ongoing national commitment to ensuring that all citizens with disabilities have access to the assistive technology they need to enjoy full and productive lives.

VERMONT ASSISTIVE TECHNOLOGY PROJECT: PROJECT ACCOMPLISHMENTS

- In collaboration with VR and DET, made all twelve DET sites technologically accessible to Vermonters with disabilities seeking employment
- Established demo and tryout centers for adapted computers, augmentative communication devices, software, and AT for folks with vision and hearing impairments. Leads to better buying decisions by consumers, agencies, and schools, saves money.
- 171 Vermonters (in 6 years) got the loans they needed to purchase AT through the Adaptive Equipment Revolving Fund.
- Prescription to delivery time for new wheelchairs has been cut in half.
- Over 50,000 Vermonters have received training in availability of, access to, and use of appropriate assistive technology.
- The recycle catalog enables consumers to recycle used AT. Lowers costs.
- The "How Do I Pay For It?" funding guide enables consumers to navigate the systems (both public and private) that fund AT. Over 8,000 distributed.
- Developed and support the Rehabilitation Engineering Technician Program at VTC. Results in better qualified technicians providing service to consumers through agencies, non-profits, vendors, and schools. Only program of its type in the nation.
- Supports the Independent (a newspaper) providing information about AT to over 15,000 elders and people with disabilities.
- Enabled agencies such as VCIL, VPIC, and the AAA's to deliver effective information and referral services pertaining to AT.
- Thousands of Vermonters have been able to see, touch, and talk about AT at numerous technology fairs and recreation expos. Leads to better buying decisions.
- Collaborative partner with Departments of Education, Employment and Training, Voc-Rehab, and other state agencies. Provide the support and information necessary to enable these agencies to integrate AT policy into their work.
- Have recently formed a non-profit to address ongoing AT needs cross-age and cross-disability. Potential activities of the non-profit include: used equipment recycling on a much larger scale than the current effort, a lending library of AT for schools, regional demo and tryout centers, AT training, and information and referral.

Rehabilitation Engineering Technology

Helping People Through Technology

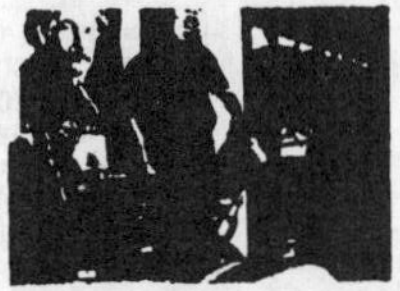

Technology is advancing so rapidly it seems almost daily that another breakthrough promises to change forever some aspect of our lives. For people with disabilities, that promise is already being fulfilled – with profound impact.

Computers can now give voice to thoughts once silenced by injury or illness... "smart" mechanical devices can compensate for nerves or muscles that no longer respond... high-tech electronics translates speech to the written word, and vice-versa... improvements in orthopedic and prosthetic devices from wheelchairs to artificial limbs have brought vast improvements in mobility, independence, and job opportunities for people with disabilities.

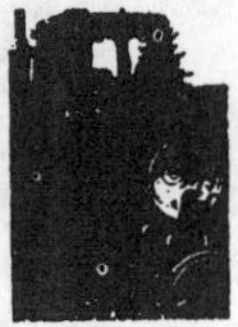

Rehabilitation Engineering is the professional discipline given to adapting today's new technologies to assist people with disabilities. Vermont Tech's two-year degree program in Rehabilitation Engineering Technology prepares students as technicians skilled in delivering these rehabilitation engineering services.

Working with a rehabilitation team, rehabilitation engineering technicians assess needs, identify problems, and devise solutions based on available assistive technology. Depending on the needs of the individual, the technician might be called on to modify commercially-available devices or to build customized devices that meet special needs.

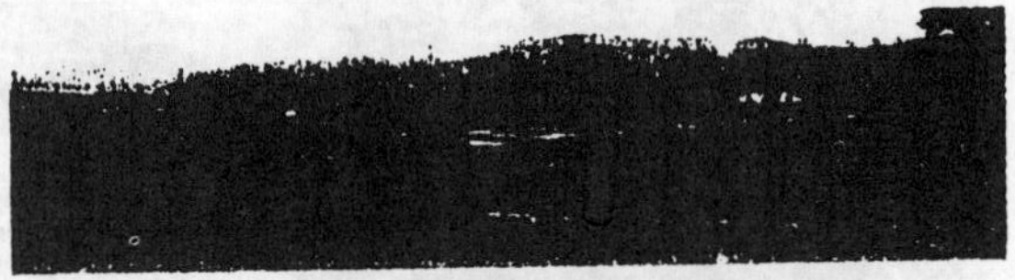

Scholarship Opportunities

The Rehabilitation Engineering Technology program is funded in part by the Rehabilitation Services Administration (RSA). Between their first and second years, students are given the option of participating in a 10-week summer internship at a rehabilitation facility. Students who participate in the internship receive a $3000 stipend from RSA. Possible internship sites include, but are not limited to: Crotched Mountain Rehabilitation Center (NH); Helen Hayes Hospital (NY); Vermont Rehabilitation Engineering Center; Vermont Association for the Blind and Visually Impaired; and Vermont Vocational Rehabilitation. The six seniors with the highest grade point averages are offered an RSA Training Stipend of $4000 in their senior year to be used for tuition, books, and travel to a rehabilitation engineering conference.

Program Overview

The interdisciplinary Rehabilitation Engineering Technology program combines traditional courses in mechanical and electrical engineering, mathematics, physics, and language arts with specialized courses in assistive technology and disabilities. Throughout the program, students have frequent opportunities to interact with consumers of assistive technology and with professionals who provide services to them.

Career Opportunities

Rehabilitation engineering technicians work in a wide range of occupations in vocational, medical, and educational settings. Rehabilitation hospitals, vocational training centers, rehabilitation research centers, assistive technology manufacturers, medical equipment sales, and public and private agencies all need rehabilitation engineering technicians. Recent graduates are employed by durable medical equipment dealers as wheelchair seating specialists, by rehabilitation research centers as adaptive computer specialists, and by vocational training centers as computer access training specialists.

Curriculum

First Year

Fall

- MA 102 Technical Mathematics (4)
- PH 101 Physics I (4)
- GE 104 Literature and Composition (3)
- EL 115 General Electronics I (4)
- CS 108 Computer Software and Programming (2)
- RT 161 Freshman Seminar (0)

Spring

- MA 106 Calculus (4)
- PH 110 Physics II (4)
- EL 116 General Electronics II (4)
- MT 105 Manufacturing Processes (3)
- MT 111 Mechanical Drafting (1)
- RT 233 Disabilities Studies (3)

Second Year

Fall

- MT 203 Applied Mechanics (3)
- MT 2[illegible] Mechanisms (3)
- EL 241 Digital Systems (4)
- RT 201 Architectural Drafting (1)
- GE 106 Technical Communication (3)
- GE XXX General Education Elective (3)

Spring

- EL 244 Electronic Applications (4)
- MT 204 Strength of Materials (3)
- RT 244 Mechanical and Home Modifications (3)
- RT 228 Computer Modifications (3)
- GE XXX General Education Elective (3)

Regional Student Program Offers Reduced Tuition.

The Regional Student Program makes it possible for many New England students to enroll in the Rehabilitation Engineering Technology program at a tuition rate substantially below the Vermont non-resident rate. Call Admissions for details.

Admissions Procedures

Applicants to the Rehabilitation Engineering Technology associate's degree program should have completed Algebra I & II, Geometry and Laboratory Physics in high school, in addition to the English and history/social science normally required for high school graduation. A completed VTC application, secondary school transcripts, letters of recommendation, and SAT or ACT scores should be forwarded to the Admissions Office.

Applications and Admissions Questions
Admissions Office
Vermont Technical College
Randolph Center VT 05061
802-728-1243 or
800-442-8821
(Northeastern U.S.)
Email:
admissions@night.vtc.vsc.edu
World Wide Web:
http://www.vtc.vsc.edu

Come for a Visit

To learn more about this program and about Vermont Tech, you are invited to visit. Tour the campus with a student guide. Talk with our admissions and financial aid staff. Meet faculty members from the program area. Tours and interviews are generally available weekdays during the school year, but arrangements can be made for Saturday and summer visits.

For an Appointment Call:

Weekdays, 8 a.m. to 4:30 p.m.
(802) 728-1243 (Voice/TDD) or
(800) 442-8821 (Voice/TDD in Northeastern U.S.)

Nondiscrimination Policy
The Vermont State Colleges comply with state and federal laws related to equal opportunity and non-discrimination. Qualified students are recruited for, admitted to, and participate in all college programs without discrimination on the basis of race, color, sex, sexual orientation, religion, creed, national origin, age, veteran status, or disability. The Vermont State Colleges will provide reasonable accommodations to

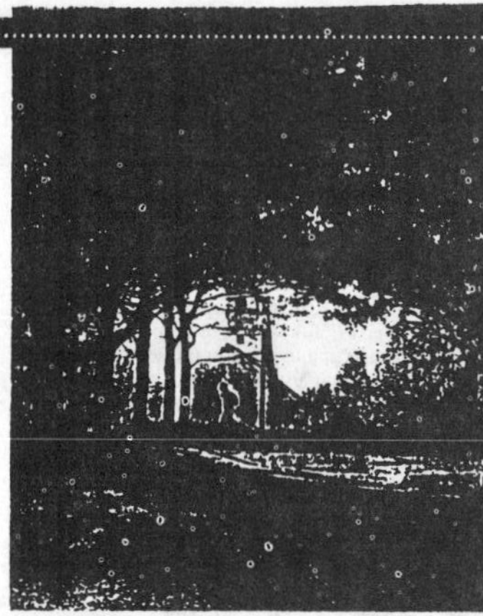

About Vermont Tech

Vermont Technical College is a public college offering 17 associate's and bachelor's degrees in technology-related fields. The 700-student institution is part of the five-member Vermont State Colleges system. Vermont Tech is located on a 544-acre campus in the village of Randolph Center, Vermont, 1 mile east of exit 4 of Interstate 89. The College has maintained an enviable placement record—98% since 1982. The 1-to-13 faculty-to-student ratio ensures that students get the individual attention they need in order to succeed.

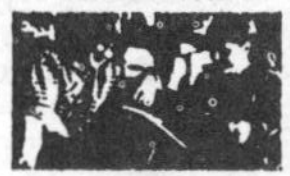

VERMONT TECHNICAL COLLEGE

COME FOR A VISIT

RANDOLPH CENTER, VT 05061
800-442-VTC-1
admissions@night.vtc.vsc.edu

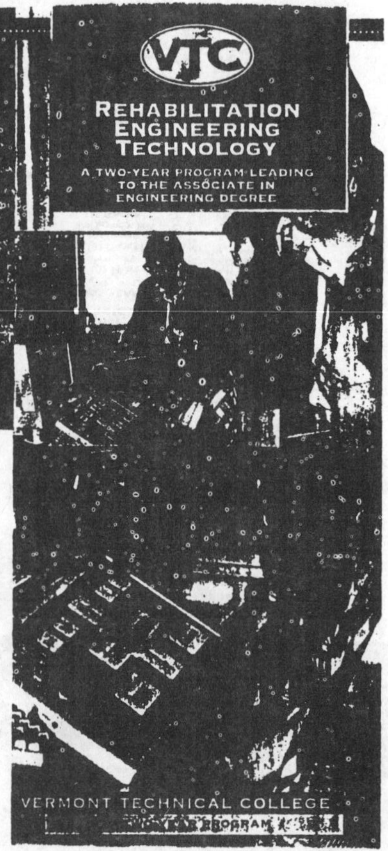

The CHAIRMAN. Mr. Pawlek.

Mr. PAWLEK. Thank you, Senator Jeffords.

I would like to thank you for this opportunity to speak on assistive technology-related issues.

The design of the Tech Act allows each State to address the needs of its own citizens in its own way. In addition to wisely spending the Federal dollars allocated to the State, the project has taken steps to establish partnerships and collaborative relationships that will enhance the effectiveness of the program and expand resources available to individuals with disabilities. An area in which we have achieved a great deal of success is in developing partnerships with the private sector.

One of these private sector relationships is illustrated in the development of our Recycled Equipment Marketplace, the REM.

The New Hampshire model is built on the principles of a free marketplace and focuses on using medical equipment vendors as the primary distribution system for used equipment. Vendors can purchase at very low cost devices that have been donated to the REM from a variety of sources, including manufacturers, health care facilities and individuals. The result is a lower-cost alternative to meet the needs of individuals who have no insurance coverage, individuals who have limited insurance coverage, or individuals who for their own purposes choose a lower-cost alternative. They system that has been developed includes all citizens, basically.

In the first 3 years of operation of this program, over 4,000 individuals in New Hampshire have accessed this program, with nearly 2,000 items being brought into the system and 1,200 pieces going out. Through this process, we estimate that $500,000 in savings to New Hampshire health care consumers has resulted. In the current year, sales have increased significantly, creating increased savings to consumers and, most importantly, has moved the program very close to reaching its goal of self-sufficiency. The possibilities for health care savings in the long run are tremendous.

In an effort to make information about this program as well as other equipment distribution programs available to more individuals, a related private sector development has been the creation of an interactive web site for equipment exchange. In collaboration with a major internet provider, the Yuri Rubinsky Foundation, and the other five New England States, an exciting new resource is currently available. The web site allows individuals or organizations to list or search for equipment that is available for sale, loan or donation, thus providing greater expansion of the ability to reuse devices. Again, through memberships and private sector advertising, the system will be self-sustaining.

In related activity, we have been able to develop relationships with organizations around the world to move our surplus items to places such as the Dominican Republic, China, Bosnia, Pakistan and Poland. And in a tribute to one of your Senate colleagues, Senator Bob Smith of New Hampshire last year assisted in delivering equipment to Poland while on another mission.

Another project in the area of private sector collaboration is the development of low-interest loan guarantee programs. Our is in conjunction with one of our statewide banks, the Bank of New

Hampshire. As Judy Heumann mentioned this morning, there are 36 States that also have similar financial programs for loans. Through this program, individuals who have an assistive technology need can borrow up to $5,000 to purchase computers, do housing modifications, install a lift in a van, or purchase adapted recreation equipment. These are uses for which there is typically no other funding source available.

Because this is a loan program, it is available to individuals from all income levels and promotes the concept that personal investment in the program will help to ensure the system is more responsive to individual needs.

These activities and others are designed to become part of the infrastructure supporting access to assistive technology. These programs have the effect of relieving pressure on other programs such as Medicaid, vocational rehabilitation and schools. The fact that they are designed to become self-sustaining make their value even more apparent.

Other project-supported activities such as information and referral, training, and awareness programs, while also helping to relieve pressure on elements of State and local governments, are much more difficult to get to the point of self-sufficiency. The economic dynamics of the internet is changing some of those perspectives, but there is still a long way to go to get cash-strapped governmental organizations to support the flow of usable information and training.

My recommendations for future legislation focus on supporting the types of activities that I have described. First, I feel that it is important to support projects in all States. Each State is unique and will develop its own solutions to problems as well as set its own priorities as to the problems it wants to address.

The design of the Tech Act has been such that there is the flexibility for each State to define its priorities and develop creative solutions to meet assistive technology needs. The programs that I have mentioned are products of this system, and there are many more success stories throughout the country.

Second, I would recommend that there be support for initiatives that have proven themselves effective. Through the process of developing statewide initiatives, projects that have the potential of national significance have been identified and should be expanded. Programs such as the equipment recycling program, loan programs and many others have worked well in States, and support for their replication should be provided.

At a regional forum on assistive technology held last month in Boston, a medical equipment company owner was asked how to further stimulate private sector involvement in assistive technology programs. His answer was to support the expansion of successful programs developed in conjunction with private sector input, and let the marketplace take its course.

With that, I would like to again thank you for this opportunity and look forward to supporting new legislation that will expand access to assistive technologies for all persons with disabilities.

The CHAIRMAN. Thank you for your very helpful testimony.

[The prepared statement of Mr. Pawlek follows:]

PREPARED STATEMENT OF MARION J. PAWLEK

I would like to thank the committee for this opportunity to speak on assistive technology related issues. My name is Marion Pawlek and I have been coordinating the Tech Act project at the University of New Hampshire's, Institute on Disability for the past seven years. Over the last 25 years, I have been involved in financial management of health care related organizations in hospital and community settings.

The design of the Tech Act allows each state to address the needs of its own citizens in its own way. In New Hampshire, we tend to look at issues conservatively and try to get the most mileage out of every dollar that is available. In addition to wisely spending the federal dollars allocated to the State, the project has taken steps to establish partnerships and collaborative relationships that will enhance the effectiveness of the program and expand the resources available to individuals with disabilities. An area in which we have achieved a great deal of success is in developing partnerships with the private sector.

One of these private sector relationships is illustrated in the development of our Recycled Equipment Marketplace (REM). There are many well intentioned programs around the country that are designed to reuse medical equipment by giving items to individuals who have needs. These programs must rely on federal, state, private sources to maintain their programs and usually only provide service to individuals with limited means.

The New Hampshire model is built on the principles of the free marketplace and focuses on using medical equipment vendors the primary distribution system for used equipment. Vendors can purchase, at very low cost, devices that have been donated to the REM from a variety of sources including manufacturers, health care facilities, and individuals. The result is a lower cost alternative to meet needs for individuals who have no insurance coverage, individuals who have limited insurance coverage, or individuals who for their own purposes choose a lower cost alternative. Thus a system that includes all citizens has been created.

In the first three years of operation, over 4000 individuals in New Hampshire have accessed this program with nearly 2000 items being brought into the system and 1200 pieces going out. Through this process, we estimate that $500,000 in savings to New Hampshire health care consumers has resulted. In the current year, sales have increased significantly creating increased savings to consumers and most importantly, has moved the program very close to reaching its goal of self sufficiency. Imagine the possibilities for health care cost savings if this program were initiated on a national level.

In an effort to make information about this program, as well as other equipment distribution programs available to more individuals, a related private sector development has been the creation of an interactive web site for equipment exchange. In collaboration with a major internet provider, the Yuri Rubinsky Foundation, and the other five New England states, an exciting new resource is currently available. The web site allows individuals or organizations to list or search for equipment that is available for sale, loan, or donation thus providing for a greater expansion of the ability to reuse devices. Again, through memberships and private sector advertising, the system will be self-sustaining.

In related activity, we have been able to develop relationships with organizations around the world to move our surplus items to places such as the Dominican Republic, China, Bosnia, Pakistan, and Poland. We have developed a working arrangement with Puerto Rico for the ongoing transfer of equipment. And in a tribute to another of your senate colleagues, Senator Bob Smith of New Hampshire last year assisted in delivering equipment to Poland while on another mission. The press coverage from both New Hampshire and the village in Poland where the equipment was sent are attached to your packet.

Another project in the area of private sector collaboration is the development of a low interest loan guarantee program in conjunction with one of our statewide banks, the Bank of New Hampshire. There are currently 21 states that also have some form of financial loan program available. Through this program, individuals who have an assistive technology need can borrow up to $5,000 to purchase computers, do housing modifications, install a lift in a van, or purchase adapted recreation equipment. These are uses for which there is typically no other funding source available. Because this is a loan program, it is available to individuals from all income levels and promotes the concept that personal investment in a program will help to insure the system is more responsive to individual needs.

The Bank of New Hampshire, as part of its community reinvestment responsibility, has actively joined this partnership and provides all of its administrative services at no cost . In addition, the interest rates are kept at 1 percent to 2 percent which makes loans much more affordable. The bank clearly sees the long term benefits of involvement both from the public benefit view of doing the right thing, and being involved in a program that will provide for development of long term relationships that will be good for business.

These activities, and others, are designed to become part of the infrastructure supporting access to assistive technology. These programs have the effect of relieving pressure on other programs such as Medicaid, vocational rehabilitation, and schools. The fact that they are designed to become self-sustaining make their value even more apparent.

Other project supported activities such as Information and referral, training, and awareness programs, while also helping to relieve pressure on elements of state and local governments, are much more difficult to get to the point of self-sufficiency. Many organizations, in their own attempts to be cost conscious, are reluctant to pay for these types of activities. The internet is changing some of that perspective, but there is still a long way to go in getting cash strapped governmental organizations to support the flow of useable information and training.

My recommendations for future legislation focus on supporting the type of activities that I have described. First, I feel that it is important to support projects in all states. Each state is unique and will develop its own solutions to problems as well as set its own priorities as to the problems it wants to address. The design of the Tech Act has been such that there is the flexibility for each state to define its priorities and develop creative solutions to meet assistive technology needs. The programs that I have mentioned are products of this system and there are many more success stories throughout the country.

Secondly, I would recommend that there be support for initiatives that have proven themselves effective. Through the process of developing statewide initiatives, projects that have the potential of national significance have been identified and should be expanded. Programs such as the equipment recycling program, loan programs and many others have worked well in states and support for their replication should be provided. At a regional forum on assistive technology held last month in Boston, a medical equipment company owner was asked how to further stimulate private sector involvement in assistive technology programs. His answer was to support the expansion of successful programs developed in conjunction with private sector input and let the marketplace take its course.

Again, I would like to thank the chairman for the opportunity to address the committee and look forward to supporting new legislation that will expand the access to assistive technology for all persons with disabilities.

Senator's Search for MIAs Takes Him t

By MICHAEL COUSINEAU
Union Leader Staff

Sen. Bob Smith's hunt for answers on missing American servicemen in Vietnam took him to Russia where he heard a military doctor recall how he talked to a wounded American soldier in Vietnam more than 20 years ago.

"It was a very touching story that he offered a bit of kindness to a prisoner of war," Smith said by phone from Warsaw, Poland, yesterday."

"He told us he saw him and spoke to him," the New Hampshire Republican said. In a sign of the compassion the doctor showed, Smith said, "The doctor asked, if he's alive he would like to speak to him."

No one knows whether the badly wounded soldier recovering in a Hanoi hospital made it back home, but Smith said his current weeklong trip to Russia, Poland and the Czech Republic as part of a U.S.-Russian commission will hopefully find a few more answers.

"We found a little new information, but not a lot," said Smith, a crusader on resolving the fate of unaccounted for soldiers.

The search will be measured in inches — not miles.

"It's a tedious process, but we try to piece together what we can," Smith said. "I'm somewhat disappointed we didn't get more information."

Smith's plane also carried medical supplies — including wheelchairs and incubators — that Tamworth resident Margo Maller organized. The supplies came from Memorial Hospital in North Conway and the New Hampshire Alliance of Assistive Technology, which has a partnership with a hospital in Krotoszyn, Poland.

"These are the types of things that are not common here," he said. "We had room for them and they were very appreciative."

Those supplies will reach the hospital today. The wife of U.S. Ambassador to Poland Nicholas Rey coincidentally met Maller recently and the ambassador thanked Smith for the supplies.

The compassionate doctor was among 21 Russian veterans who served in Vietnam and talked to the group. Many of them manned anti-aircraft artillery or missile sites. They offered some information on U.S. planes shot down.

Smith al
that contai
sonal effect
U.S. service

The com
cials. In Po
Poles who

Each per
nam may
whereabou

Smith, a
Committee
Czech Rep
to archive
President
The trip m

KROTOSZYŃSKA

Wtorek 29 lipca 1997 Nr 25/1997/2046-1 Nr indeksu 348 120 ISSN 0208-7421 cena 50 gr

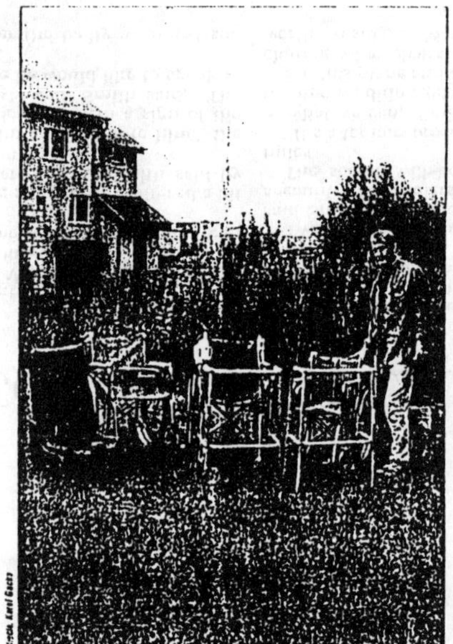

Zdjęcie Karol Gacza

Mirosław Korcz prezentuje dary od Amerykanów.

Dar z Ameryki

Nazwisko Margo Mallar kojarzy się krotoszynianom przede wszystkim z letnią szkołą języka angielskiego, którą prowadzi ze swymi przyjaciółmi od paru lat. Margo postanowiła jednak nie poprzestać na działalności edukacyjnej.

Przy pomocy wielu organizacji i ludzi dobrej woli, zajęła się organizowaniem pomocy dla miejscowej służby zdrowia oraz Stowarzyszenia na Rzecz Dzieci i Osób Niepełnosprawnych. Organizacja ta przed kilkoma miesiącami otrzymała dwa wózki dla małych dzieci. Kolejne dary przybyły do Krotoszyna w lipcu.

Do Polski dostarczył je (specjalnym samolotem wojskowym) senator Bob Smith, który przybył do Warszawy w poszukiwaniu wieści o losach jeńców amerykańskich w Wietnamie. Senator jest człowiekiem znanym ze swej dobroczynnej działalności. Z darami i pomocą docierał już do wielu rejonów świata, m in. do Bośni.

Tym razem przywiózł przesyłkę od *N.H. Alliance for Assistive Technology*. Jest to społeczna organizacja, która zajmuje się renowacją sprzętu szpitalnego i rehabilitacyjnego oraz przekazywaniem go tam, gdzie jest potrzebny. W ten właśnie sposób do Krotoszyna trafiły dwa pionizatory, trzy wózki młodzieżowe, chodziki i krzesełka do karmienia dzieci niesiedzących, balkoniki i inne urządzenia.

Fundacja Margo o nazwie *World News Crews* przekazała sprzęt stowarzyszeniu, którego członkami są przede wszystkim rodzice dzieci niepełnosprawnych. Jego prezes - Mirosław Korcz powiedział „ZK", że sprzęt jest bardzo przydatny i trafi we właściwe ręce. Na razie część darów znajduje się w punkcie rehabilitacyjnym. Większość otrzymają przedszkola integracyjne (nr 6 i 7).

Rok temu - za pośrednictwem *Rotary Club* i fundacji M. Mallar - jeden ze szpitali przekazał miejscowej lecznicy aparat EKG.

Wkrótce do New Hampshire wyjedzie grupa stażystów. Jednym z nich jest krotoszyniak, absolwent gdańskiej AWF - Maciej Blandzi. Będzie on praktykował w klinice rehabilitacyjnej pod egidą *N.H. Allianse For Assistive Technology*.

Maciej stanie się dla nas łącznikiem między Polską i Ameryką. Ma dobrą orientację w tym, co tutaj może się przydać - powiedziała Margo. *Mam też nadzieję, że zdobyte w USA doświadczenia przeniosą na polski grunt*

UNIVERSITY OF NEW HAMPSHIRE

Institute on Disability
Assistive Technology Partnership Project
The Concord Center, Suite 307
10 Ferry St., Unit #14
Concord, New Hampshire 03301-5019

Tel: (603)224-0630 (V/TDD)
In NH (800)427-3338 (V/TDD)
FAX: (603) 228-3270

Marion Pawlek

Marion is currently the project coordinator for the New Hampshire Tech Act program, the Assistive Technology Partnership Project located at the University of New Hampshire's, Institute on Disability. He has been with the project since its inception in 1992. During this time, many initiatives have been undertaken including the development of non-profit organizations, training programs, the development of an information and referral system, the development of a financial loan program, and the development of a very comprehensive equipment recycling program, as well as involvement with many technology related policy initiatives.

Marion has presented extensively around the country on assistive technology related issues including equipment reuse, recycling, and corporate development for achieving financial independence. In addition. he has consulted with many states on related issues and has developed ongoing relationships throughout the country and territories.

Prior, to working on this project, for 10 years, Marion was president of a company doing financial management for community organizations specializing in the areas of mental health and developmental services. For the seven years prior, he was assistant director of patient accounting at New Hampshire's largest hospital, the Dartmouth Hitchcock Medical Center.

Marion received his undergraduate degree at Colby College in Waterville Maine in 1972, and earned his MBA from Plymouth State College in Plymouth, New Hampshire in 1994.

Marion is married to Cynthia who is a reference librarian at Dartmouth College and has two daughters Sarah who is a freshman at Vassar College in Poughkeepsie N.Y., and Chelsea who is a sophomore in high school.

Resources for Independence

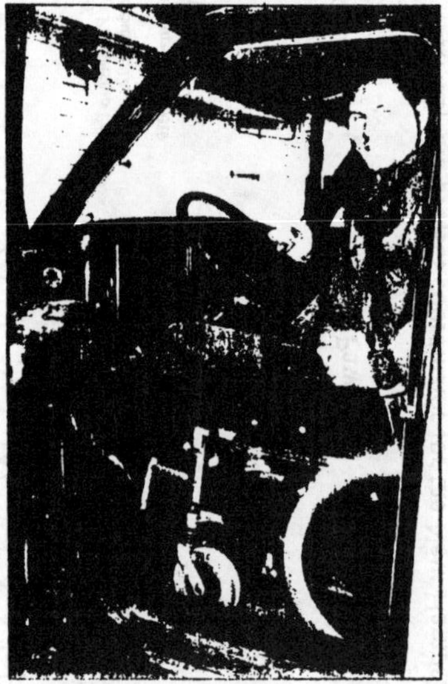

"Because of assistive technologies I am able to lead an independent life." – Jim Sullivan

There's a Bank of New Hampshire Office Near You!

Allenstown	485-4011
Barrington	664-5800
Bristol	744-8521
Concord	225-4500
Contoocook	746-4121
Dover	742-2100
Epsom	736-9363
Goffstown	497-6000
Hampton	926-6868
Hillsborough	464-5527
Hooksett	668-2192
Hudson	880-5400
Manchester	624-6600
Merrimack	880-5400
Nashua	880-5400
Newmarket	659-6746
Northwood	942-8739
Portsmouth	433-4320
Suncook	485-9564

Assistive Technology Loans

a low-interest loan program
to help promote independent living
through assistive devices
and related services,
or modifications for accessibility.

BANK OF NEW HAMPSHIRE

in collaboration with:
New Hampshire Alliance for Assistive Technology,
UNH/UAP New Hampshire Assistive
Technology Partnership Project and
Southeastern Regional Education Service Center

Equipment for Independent Living

Working Together for Independence

The New Hampshire Alliance for Assistive Technology (NHAAT), UNH/UAP New Hampshire Assistive Technology Partnership Project (NHATPP), Southeastern Regional Education Service Center (SERESC), and Bank of New Hampshire have joined together to provide low interest loans for acquiring assistive technology.

What is Assistive Technology?

Assistive Technology Device

Any piece of equipment or product which increases, maintains or improves functional capabilities of an individual with a disability.

Assistive Technology Service

Any service that directly assists an individual with a disability in the selection, acquisition or use of an assistive technology device.

Assistive technology devices and services can increase independence, productivity, self-worth and integration at home, school or in the workplace. Examples include:

- Modified computers
- Walkers, scooters and wheelchairs
- Communication boards
- Environmental control systems
- Adapted recreational equipment
- Home/work site modifications

The Loan Program

Who is eligible?

Any New Hampshire resident or parent/guardian of a New Hampshire resident with a physical or mental impairment that substantially limits one or more major life activities.

What can the loan be used for?

Any assistive technology, equipment or related services, used to improve an individual's independence or to assist them in becoming more productive members of the community.

How much can be borrowed?

Loans of $1,000 to $5,000 are available. The loan term may be from one to five years. The interest rate will be established at the time of application and will be fixed for the entire term. The rate will be a special discounted rate based on the current rate for regular savings accounts.

How are the decisions made?

Loans are considered on the basis of:

- your completed application
- selection of appropriate equipment and training
- financial status and credit history

How to apply:

Visit any of the 29 Bank of New Hampshire offices for an application, or call NHAAT at 1-800-427-3338 to request one.

SERESC
Southeastern Regional Education Service Cente
"A non-profit educational collaborative providing q
services to public schools"
11 Peabody Road, Derry, NH 03038
603-434-0556

NHAAT
New Hampshire Alliance for Assistive Techno
"Increasing access to and availability
of assistive technology"
The Concord Center, Suite 321, 10 Ferry Stree
Unit #25, Concord, NH 03301-5081
Laconia, NH 03247
603-228-2088/800-427-3338 (V/TTY)

NHATPP
NH Assistive Technology Partnership Proje
UNH, Institute on Disability/UAP
"Improving the quality of life for people in NH
through assistive technology"
The Concord Center, Suite 307, 10 Ferry Stee
Unit #14, Concord, NH 03301-5019
603-224-0630/800-427-3338 (V/TTY)

BANK OF NEW HAMPSHIRE
Equal Opportunity Lender

The Loan Fund Program provided by the NHAAT in conjunction with a Federal Grant from NIDRR and the Guaranteed Collateral Loan Program, is funded by SERESC through the Bank of New Hampshire.

The CHAIRMAN. Craig, please proceed.

Mr. FULFORD. Thank you for allowing me this opportunity to speak before you. I have cerebral palsy, which resulted in physical, visual and learning disabilities. I would like to show you now how assistive technology helps me and would help other individuals in their lives.

[Demonstration of Intellitalk Program]: Welcome to the world of assistive technology. This talking world processing program manufactured by Intellitools, called Intellitalk, will read by letter, word, sentence, paragraph or the entire document, and it only costs $39.95. All we have done to this laptop is put in a sound card and added a software program to make this accessible for me.

I use more sophisticated pieces of assistive technology on my personal computer in my dorm room. I use high- and low-tech devices. When I am preparing for a test, I scan in class notes and terms into a scanner which converts the material to Word and reads it to me. the laptop, scanner, Openbook software and Dec talk were jointly funded by education and vocational rehabilitation services and exited with me when I left high school. My other pieces of assistive technology were purchased by mom and dad.

I have made some hard choices in my life already. Receiving an education was so important to me that Mom and I left my father, grandfather and friends in rural southwestern Indiana to attend Lawrence North High School in Indianapolis. It was hard to go from a self-contained classroom to all general education classes with the use of assistive technology, but I did it. I was active in chorus and participated on the speech team. I graduated 138 out of 401. I am very proud of my accomplishments.

I am finishing my freshman year at Vincennes University carrying a gradepoint average of 2.9. I am enrolled in the Business Studies Options program and will be enrolling in the assistive technology degree program next year. My vocational goal is to become a qualified assistive technology provider.

This all sounds like this has been so simple, but it has not. Getting to this point has been and continues to be a struggle. Accessibility is a barrier in all areas of my life. Educational programs, building structures, sidewalks, transportation, and even accessible technology is doable, but not readily accessible.

As you begin to decide about assistive technology, please provide the resources for direct access to assistive technology for consumers. Tech Act programs have helped a lot of people.

Thank you for this opportunity. It has been an honor to share my assistance technology and thoughts.

The CHAIRMAN. Thank you, Craig. That was very helpful, and I appreciate you being here. This hearing today has been very, very helpful to all of us and those who are watching on television to better understand what this bill is all about and the necessity to continue it and hopefully improve it. I would like to ask a couple of questions about what we need to do to improve it or, in any event, to continue it.

I am sorry—Ms. Fulford. Craig gave such eloquent testimony, I did not realize you would be supplementing it.

Ms. Fulford. That is okay. He is a hard act to follow, I am telling you; he is so good.

Mr. FULFORD. With the help of the laptop, of course.

The CHAIRMAN. Right, and excuse me. Please go ahead.

Ms. Fulford. ATTAIN began in July of 1990. Consistent with congressional intent, ATTAIN is a consumer-responsive, consumer-driven assistive technology project based on the identified needs of consumers through annual statewide needs assessments, focus groups and town meetings.

The principal needs of Indiana, according to the 1997 findings, are: 1) more assistive technology service providers; 2) more qualified personnel to assess assistive technology to assure the most appropriate devices selected by the consumer which reduces inaccurate purchases and abandonment of devices; 3) more training to increase the knowledge and skill level of consumers and services providers.

ATTAIN's response to these identified needs has been a two-pronged approach. One is a systems change team composed of consumers, ATTAIN, protection and advocacy, State agencies and other disability organizations to alleviate statewide barriers impacting assistive technology. Community technology networks work at the local level to alleviate the barrier.

To highlight just a couple of ATTAIN's accomplishments, we have developed a buyout methodology. This is a formula that calculates the cost depreciation of devices when infants and toddlers and children and students with disabilities are transitioning from early intervention to education and education to vocational rehabilitation services. Medicaid codes were changed to be more specific for the timely acquisition of augmentative alternative communication devices.

The second approach is education and training. Team assessment modules targeting the life span are being implemented. All four modules contain assessment profile forms to guide a consumer-driven team through the assistive technology selection process. ATTAIN trains consumers and service providers about the laws and regulations regarding assistive technology. These trainers provide training in their local communities. ATTAIN has hosted numerous statewide and local conferences and workshops.

Establishing statewide partnerships is necessary and highly effective because most of Indiana is rural, with distinctly different cultures based upon geography. This is true throughout many of the Tech Act States.

We understand the unique characteristics of the people and the communities within the State. Governor O'Bannon has made it a priority for all programs serving the same population to coordinate services to meet the needs of consumers. Our activities would not have been successful if ATTAIN had attempted to address the issues in a vacuum.

Interstate informal agreements have been reached with Kentucky and Ohio, allowing consumers to cross the border, reaching any city that they need to in order to access assistive technology. Current formal contracts with ATTAIN are with the independent living center, the AGR-Ability Project in Indiana, and Protection and Advocacy; and I have provided more in my written testimony.

You have asked me to speak about the Indiana Certificate Program. ATTAIN initiated the assistive technology degree program by providing a grant to Vincennes University to work with other universities statewide to develop and integrate an assistive technology curriculum into postsecondary education. Under the continued leadership of Governor O'Bannon, a brand new educational program targeting undergraduates has been developed. These programs will prepare students with the knowledge and skills to provide a practical approach to assistive technology applications in education, rehabilitation, health care, business, and other related settings.

The certificate program will increase professional development for individuals with experience in assistive technology or those with degrees in related fields. Upon completion of the associate's degree program, the student will be prepared for a career in assistive technology. Both programs will complement the formal certification and credentialing process of the assistive technology practitioners and suppliers competencies being implemented by RESNA, a national not-for-profit association concerned with rehabilitation and assistive technology services for individuals with disabilities. The goal of both programs is to increase the quality of service providers and provide assurances and safeguards for consumers.

ATTAIN continues to collaborate with Vincennes University to implement the certificate program beginning in the fall of 1998, while the associate's degree program is currently awaiting approval from the Indiana Higher Education Commission. It is our hope and expectation that the Indiana certification program can be replicated as a model throughout the United States.

You also asked me to address sustaining the infrastructure of education and employment. The factors that I believe contribute to a State's willingness to create and sustain the infrastructure include education of the needs, belief in the potential of what can be achieved and the appropriate capacity to meet the needs of people with disabilities. These are the three principal factors.

With the coming of the information highway, every school is to be wired, and every student is to have his own computer. Accessibility issues exist. The funding for educational technology has not sufficiently addressed the needs of students with disabilities. Assistive technology needs have not been included in the funding. Access to providers and especially qualified providers is an issue for consumers and State agencies purchasing assistive technology. Reporting and tracking of assistive technology purchases within State agencies for cost-saving purposes is a must.

Tech Act programs play a vital role as assistive technology experts. We represent the consumers to assure assistive technology needs are being addressed within State agency plans, regulations, policy manuals and other areas. Speaking for Indiana, utilizing the systems change and training approaches has improved access to assistive technology, but we have not achieved the quality provider capacity nor have we done what I call institutionalizing the issues around assistive technology into the day-to-day decisionmaking of our schools or our employers.

State agencies such as education and vocational rehabilitation have made progress toward meeting the needs of consumers regarding assistive technology, but institutionalization is still a far reach. Providing funds for State agencies to purchase assistive technology is just as important as continuing the Tech Act programs and programs such as IDEA, the Rehab Act and others.

Strides have been made. We are at a more in-depth level than we were in 1994. Other factors such as managed care are impacting assistive technology, and much work remains to be done. Without continued Federal support, it will be difficult to ensure that accessibility, systems change, education, training, and developing the capacity to provide quality assistive technology devices and services will occur.

In most cases, consumers are not asking for something unique and totally different. Having access to the same technology everyone else has increases independence and productivity of consumers tenfold. Without the expertise that has been and continues to be developed through the Tech Act, a great opportunity will be lost to truly allow individuals with disabilities to live, work and succeed.

My personal experiences, my professional goals are all contained within my materials. I think that what Craig in his testimony is trying to tell you is that, yes, the world is changing, but there are still many things that need to be done for Craig and all others.

Thank you for this opportunity, and I would be glad to take any questions.

[The prepared statement of the Fulfords follow:]

PREPARED STATEMENT OF CRIS FULFORD, DIRECTOR, INDIANA TECH ACT, ATTAIN PROJECT

Chairman Jeffords, Senator Kennedy, Senator Coats and members of the committee: Thank you for this opportunity to discuss the importance of assistive technology to people with disabilities in Indiana and the exciting work that we are doing to ensure that people with disabilities can access technology that allows them to live, work and play in their local communities.

My name is Cris Fulford. I have been the director of the Indiana Tech Act project, Accessing Technology Through Awareness in Indiana, (ATTAIN), for almost six years. Most importantly, I am the mother of a young man, Craig, who has cerebral palsy and is an extensive user of assistive technology in every facet of his daily life. Craig is with me today. My comments to you encompass my professional and personal experiences.

I. THE INDIANA TECH ACT PROJECT/ATTAIN

ATTAIN began in July of 1990 in the second round of federal funding. The lead agency is the Indiana Family and Social Services Administration, Division of Disability, Aging and Rehabilitative Services (DDARS). For the past three years, Vincennes University, located in rural southwestern Indiana, has served as the fiscal agent for the majority of the federal Tech Act dollars.

Consistent with Congressional intent, ATTAIN is designed to meet the specific needs of Hoosiers with disabilities. Our objective is to create a consumer driven, consumer responsive, assistive technology service delivery system. Over the past seven years ATTAIN responded to consumer needs by providing information, awareness, and training. Through current needs assessments, focus groups, and town meetings statewide to gather input from individuals with disabilities, their families, representatives, state agency staff and service providers, consumers have identified the following principle needs for Indiana:

1) More assistive technology service providers qualified to do assistive technology evaluations or assessments. Although ATTAIN has contracted with several entities to increase the number of service providers, these numbers have not been able to keep up with the demands of people with disabilities.

2) More qualified personnel to evaluate and train consumers. Not only do we not have enough service providers, too many times the assessments are being done by people who are not trained. Vendors are recommending the devices they sell instead

of allowing consumers to have options and choices on what other devices might better meet their needs.

3) Reducing inaccurate purchases and abandonment of devices, which wastes money and results in consumer dissatisfaction. 27% of individuals purchase their own assistive technology in Indiana. State agencies such as the Department of Education and the Vocational Rehabilitation program purchase the bulk of devices. If the device is not appropriate, or does not fit the consumer properly, the state agency has to purchase another device, doubling the cost.

4) More training, so the State can increase the knowledge and skill level of consumers and service providers from early intervention through aging impacting assistive technology.

ATTAIN has been effective in responding to these identified needs as well as to the priorities of the Technology Related Assistance Act. The program has adopted a two-pronged approach to address the issues impacting the timely acquisition of appropriate assistive technology devices and services.

The first approach is to alleviate systemic barriers to accessing assistive technology in local communities across the state. Beginning in 1995, Indiana established a Systems Change Team, which includes ATTAIN, consumers, Protection and Advocacy, and other representatives of the particular state agency where a barrier has been identified. For further information, (**Please see Attachments: which describe the year seven system's goals, objectives and the outcomes accomplished during that period**). We are currently compiling our eighth year's accomplishments into a final report. Examples of successful outcomes from the SCT include:

Early intervention program (Part C/H of IDEA).—There are 6,800 infants and toddlers with disabilities, ages 0–2, identified by the Indiana child count. Under Governor O'Bannon's leadership, Indiana has made significant strides to increase early intervention services.

- SCT worked with the First Steps task force to define "medical" versus "developmental delay" to determine who is responsible for the acquisition of AT for infants and toddlers with disabilities.

Assistive Technology for Infants and Toddlers: SCT developed a transdisciplinary team assessment module, including assistive technology assessment profile forms, to guide a team through the selection process of AT.

- Submitted assistive technology competencies to the Indiana Professional Standards Board for licensing requirements in early childhood, general and special education teachers and speech language pathologists.

Education (Part B of IDEA)—There are 117,000 students with disabilities, ages 3-21, identified by the Indiana child count.

- SCT worked with the Division of Special Education to develop guidelines for the statewide "Indiana's Statewide Test for Educational Progress" (ISTEP) to assure students with disabilities can utilize assistive technology as documented in the Individualized Education Program.
- SCT is working with Division of Special Education (DES) to define the circumstances under which case conference committees should consider recommending the assessment of student's assistive technology needs. Article 7 (Indiana law) is being changed to reflect changes in the reauthorization of IDEA.
- Two members of the SCT continue to serve on the Division of Special Education task force to develop guidelines for an alternative assessment test for students with disabilities on non-diploma tracks to assure accountability for ALL students.

Vocational Rehabilitation Services (Employment Age)!—There were 41,300 people with disabilities who received services during fiscal year 1997.

- "Buy-Out" Methodology. DDARS (lead agency), VRS and the SCT worked with the Office of Budget Management to develop a formula of cost depreciation for infants and toddlers, children and students with disabilities who are transitioning from Part C to Part B and from Part B into VRS. The goal is to increase timeliness when students transition from one program to another when the device continues to be appropriate. VRS is working with DSE to place the methodology in the "State Transition Plan Agreement". (**Please see Attachment**)
- The SCT developed a module, *Assistive Technology on the Job:* A transdisciplinary team assessment module, including assistive technology assessment profile forms, that guide a team through the selection process of AT.
- Identified and clarified situations where the Americans with Disabilities Act (ADA) or VRS is responsible for funding AT to students in post secondary schools. Information from the technical assistance project for Protection and Advocacy assisted in clarifying these situations. The article was distributed to 57 disability services in post secondary schools and VRS offices.

The second approach is education and training. ATTAIN sponsors four trainings per year to empower consumers, families and service providers about their rights to assistive technology. Community Technology Networks have been formed to train other consumers to create local systems change and access to assistive technology in their local communities. ATTAIN has hosted or co-sponsored numerous statewide conferences, topic specific trainings, and workshops for consumers, service providers or state agency staff. At the end of 1997, ATTAIN had impacted 19,850 consumers and service providers. Knowledge empowers people to make informed choices.

I understand that Tech Act projects have been criticized in public hearings across the nation for not collaborating with other partners in the state. Let me assure you that in Indiana, this is not true.

Governor O'Bannon has made it a priority for all programs serving the same population to coordinate services to ensure that the needs of the consumer are met. None of the activities that I outlined above would have been successful if ATTAIN had attempted to address the issues in a vacuum. Since the program was established, there have been close working relationships and partnering with stakeholders across Indiana, starting with consumers.

ATTAIN has been successful only because of the relationship formed with entities such as community rehabilitation programs, Indiana University, Indiana Protection and Advocacy, Indiana's agrability program through Purdue University, independent living centers, as well as schools and state agency staff. We have worked with the Division of Special Education to jointly fund projects to break down barriers.

The statewide partnerships are important because, for the most part, Indiana is a rural state with distinctly different cultures based upon geography. For example, in the southern portion of the state, outreach to consumers occurs through family and friends. In more urban portions of the state, outreach takes place through a much more formalized process. Consumer participation in the provision of services vary depending upon where they live. Tech Projects have learned to understand the unique characteristics of the people and communities within the state. The goal in Indiana as with each of the state programs is to increase access to assistive technology by working directly with consumers in local communities.

INDIANA ATTAIN'S CERTIFICATION PROGRAM

Though I could expand upon the successes of ATTAIN, I have been asked to specifically address the fact that Indiana has responded very uniquely to the identified need of a lack of qualified assistive technology providers and vendors. Indiana, under the continued leadership of Governor O'Bannon, has developed a brand new educational program targeting undergraduates. We believe strongly that to expand capacity and respond to the need for qualified providers, we have to begin at an undergraduate level.

ATTAIN collaborated with Vincennes University through a grant to work with universities statewide to develop and integrate an assistive technology curriculum into higher education. We did this by facilitating the Assistive Technology Higher Education Project, consisting of eleven of the major universities in Indiana. A consultant reviewed sixteen various assistive technology educational or training programs nationwide ranging from complete degree programs for graduate level, distance learning, in-service training, and overview courses. The result of the Assistive Technology Higher Education Project was the development of ten modules that educators could use across disciplines to educate undergraduate students about the benefits and applications of assistive technology.

ATTAIN continues to collaborate with Vincennes University to implement an assistive technology certificate program, which is beginning in the fall of 1998, and an associates degree program currently waiting approval from the Indiana Higher Education Commission. I am proud to say our fall certification class is already filled. It is certainly our hope and expectation that the Indiana certification program can be replicated as a model throughout the United States.

These programs will prepare students with the knowledge and skills to provide a practical approach to assistive technology applications in education, rehabilitation, health care, business and a variety of related settings. The certificate program is designed to serve as professional development for individuals with experience in assistive technology or those who have degrees in related fields. Upon completion of the associates program, the student will be prepared for a career in assistive technology. **(Attachments: Certificate and Associates Degree Program, and Assistive Technology Degree Brochure)**

Both of these educational programs will complement formal certification and credentialing guidelines developed by national professional organizations. The goal of the credentialing process of the Assistive Technology Practitioners and Suppliers competencies are being implemented by RESNA, a national nonprofit association concerned with rehabilitation and assistive technology services for individuals with disabilities to increase the quality of service providers and provide assurances and safeguards for consumers.

III. SUSTAINING THE INFRASTRUCTURE

The third topic I would like to address is the need to sustain and build on the current infrastructure. I commend all of you for strengthening the language in the 1992 Rehabilitation Act Amendments and the newly reauthorized Individuals with Disabilities Education Act. Under these programs, individuals, students with disabilities, and parents are more involved than ever and have increased options and choices. Both acts require consumers to be equal partners in the development of individualized plans. Both acts have emphasized the importance of assistive technology in meeting the outcomes of the individualized educational and work-related plan and require that assistive technology be considered and documented as an option where appropriate. Education and employment goals are determined on a case-by-case basis with the control at the local level.

That is where the Tech Act comes in - we are the assistive technology experts. It is our responsibility to represent the consumers in working with the state agencies who are implementing the IDEA and the Vocational Rehab programs to make sure that assistive technology is not only part of the state plan, but that students and adults in the work force actually have access to the assistive technology they need to succeed. We work with the individual communities to address the barriers to access locally. Access to assistive technology is the key, and the Tech Act program is making access a reality through the work that we do.

It is the Tech Act in part, that provides the education and training of staff in the schools who are responsible for identifying and assessing the assistive technology needs of students under IDEA. It is the Tech Act that is training providers to assess and appropriately fit assistive technologies through the Vocational Rehabilitation program, so workers can succeed in the workforce. Without enough providers, the requirements under the Rehabilitation Act and IDEA will be meaningless. Even worse, without appropriately trained providers, whatever money is spent on assistive technologies may not be spent effectively if the assistive device is not appropriate, does not fit properly, and is abandoned.

I have been asked to comment on what factors I believe contribute to a State's willingness to create and sustain the infrastructure to support access to assistive technology in education and employment settings. Education of the needs, belief in the potential of what can be achieved, and the appropriate capacity to meet the needs of individuals and students with disabilities are what I believe to be the three principle factors.

Federal dollars account for less than 10% of the cost of education for students with disabilities. The bulk of dollars available to schools to fund AT comes from state special education funding systems. Special Education has little or no data regarding the funding of assistive technology. Billions of dollars are being expended on technology for schools with the promise of every school being wired and every student having their own computer. Yet none of the funding for educational technology has sufficiently addressed the needs of students with disabilities. Access issues are just beginning to be identified as important considerations when purchasing education technology.

Consumers and Vocational Rehabilitation counselors in Indiana have identified as their barriers to assistive technology qualified providers to assess and train consumers. Also to truly address the expectation in the Rehabilitation Act for informed choice, consumers must have more options of qualified vendors. VRS purchased $6,261,247 worth of assistive technology devices or services for 3,451 VR clients. ATTAIN worked collaboratively to refine VR's report system to accurately reflect assistive technology purchases.

Speaking for Indiana, utilizing the systems change and training approaches we have improved access to assistive technology, but we have not achieved the expert provider capacity nor have we, what I call *institutionalized* the issues around assistive technology into the day to day decision-making of our schools or employers. For example, while my son Craig was in high school, he was given a laptop. However, his laptop did not include a special adaptation/device that Craig needed. Luckily, our family could afford to purchase the necessary device that enabled Craig to meet his educational goals. I will know that my job as a Tech Act Director will no longer be needed, when I have institutionalized into the daily decision making of our educators and our employers the need for assistive technology devices to accommodate, educate, and employ people with disabilities.

While I am proud of the successes we have achieved, there remains much work to be done and federal support is still needed. Without continued federal support, it will be impossible to implement the certification program to ensure that the proper infrastructure of qualified providers are available across the nation. Even in Indiana, we are still working to make sure that access to assistive technology for education and employment is available consistently on a statewide basis to those 800,000 Hoosiers who may need it. Both education and vocational rehabilitation struggle with professional development to educate staff about assistive technology. Finding release time for front line staff and large caseloads prohibit attendance at conferences and trainings. Consumers are often educating staff about the latest in assistive technology, instead of vice versa.

In addition to the need for the federal government to continue to make this a priority, assistive technology is also costly. A device can range from ten dollars to thousands of dollars depending on the level of sophistication of the needed device. Obviously, if there is not enough funding to meet the needs of people, then they may have to go without. Others may not qualify for state assistance. Providing funds for state agencies to purchase assistive technology is just as important as continuing the Tech Act programs to provide the technical assistance, education and training.

Even though Tech Act programs do not directly purchase assistive technology devices, some states have established alternative funding programs to help individuals pay for assistive technology through low interest loan programs, buy down interest, and guaranteed loans. Tech Act programs have been creative in helping education and vocational rehabilitation services increase access to computers that are already available instead of purchasing a new computer with all the bells and whistles. Consumers are not asking for something unique and totally different. They are asking for accessibility to utilize the same computer so that a person with a disability is as productive as the next.

Exciting advancements in the field of assistive technology and new programs such as managed care were not addressed when the funds became available for the Tech Act Projects. States are struggling to adapt to these changes. Indiana has responded to the impact of managed care by being involved on the Indiana Task Force on Managed Care. This task force consists of 35 different groups involved in disability related issues. Recently, the Indiana General Assembly has passed two pieces of legislation addressing grievance procedures and consumer protections.

Finally, the need for a continued federal involvement is essential because it forces coordination between federal, state and local agencies—so that we effectively use the available dollars for consumers to obtain assistive technology devices and services in their local communities. Although progress has been made, the lack of consistent practices still exist in local agencies creating problems for consumers trying to access assistive technology. Having access to assistive technology is more important than ever for consumers of all ages.. Because of the successes in this area, premature infants are able to live with modern technology, adults are able to obtain employment with the use of technology, and seniors are able to stay in their homes longer. Without the expertise that has been and continues to be developed through the Tech Act, a great opportunity will be lost to truly allow individuals with disabilities to live, work, and succeed.

IV. PERSONAL EXPERIENCE

On a personal note, along with many others, I personally have experienced the variation in services first hand. My son, Craig, spent ten years in a segregated classroom. We went through mediation and hearings to try to get the school in our home district to include Craig in general education classes with the use of assistive technology. During the first hearing, the hearing officer ordered Craig to be moved from the junior high classroom because they were not willing to provide him with the support, training or adequate devices to meet his educational goal. He proceeded on to high school where again, nothing changed. After the second mediation and going into the second hearing, we were advised to leave the school district because of the unwillingness to provide him with the appropriate services and devices to meet his educational goals.

As Craig will tell you in his testimony, HE made the decision to leave his home, his father, grandparents and friends and move 120 miles away to an urban school for the next four years because he desperately wanted an education. After carefully researching school districts, interviewing, and visiting schools, Craig chose Lawrence North in Indianapolis, a school with the basic philosophy that every student is a contributing member of our society and should be educated as such. Craig participated all four years in general education programs with the support of assistive technology and a tutor. I am very proud to say he graduated 138th out of 401! No family should have to endure this situation. Craig is with me today and with the help of assistive technology, can tell you about it himself.

Thank you again for the opportunity to testify before you. I am happy to answer any questions that you may have.

Accessing Technology Through Awareness in INdiana
1815 N. Meridian Street, Suite 200
Indianapolis, IN 46202

AUTOBIOGRAPHY
OF
CRIS FULFORD

Cris Fulford is the director of Accessing Technology Through Awareness in Indiana (ATTAIN), a federally funded technology related assistance grant for the state of Indiana. Cris has directed this five million-dollar program since 1992. Prior to joining ATTAIN, Cris worked in the field of physical therapy for six years. In addition, Cris is the mother of a twenty-two year old son with cerebral palsy who has had to challenge the system to obtain assistive technology and other services for her son. Her son is here with her today.

Cris oversees the day to day activities of the program, develops and monitors federal and state budgets, sub contractor budgets, works with the ATTAIN Advisory Board, consumers, and others to develop new programs to address the assistive technology needs of Hoosiers with disabilities, facilitates and gains the consensus of work groups, serves on committees and task forces at the national and state level.

She provides trainings, presentations and technical assistance to consumers, and service providers on a national, state and local level regarding laws, rules and regulations impacting assistive technology in the areas of early intervention, special education, vocational rehabilitation, all medical assistance programs including managed care, adult service programs including aging, and social security.

Cris has initiated and co-authored several assistive technology modules such as: *Assistive Technology for Infants and Toddlers, Education, On The Job, and for Persons Who are Elderly, Accessibility, Accommodations for Empowering Persons with Disabilities* and the *Indiana Assistive Technology Funding Guide* now in it's second edition.

Cris has collaborated closely with Vincennes University in the development and implementation of the Assistive Technology Certificate Program and the Assistive Technology Associates Degree Program.

317-921-8766 **317-921-8774 - Fax** **800-5*A*T*T*A*I*N -Toll Free (In State)**

ATTACHMENTS

ATTAIN Brochure

ATTAIN Systems Change Team Goals

Year Seven Systems Change Team (SCT) Outcomes and Statistical Report

Buy-Out Methodology

Assistive Technology Associate of Applied Science Degree Program and Assistive Technology Certificate of Program Completion

Vincennes University Assistive Technology Brochure

ATTAIN SYSTEMS CHANGE TEAM GOALS

In order to meet the federal priorities, ATTAIN concentrates efforts in two areas: First and foremost, is the empowerment of individuals with disabilities to gain independence and actively participate in community, educational, recreational and vocational activities through the use of assistive technology. This occurs through the many training and technical assistance opportunities that ATTAIN and affiliated personnel conduct.

The second focus is to affect systems change. Systems change begins with awareness, awareness leads to information, information becomes knowledge and knowledge leads to working with others to bring about long term changes. The "Systems Change Team Goals" are the systemic efforts of the "Systems Change Team" (SCT). The team has worked diligently to collaborate with state agencies in which the barriers have been identified to alleviate the impediment to assistive technology. To date, the team has been most successful in the early childhood program, First Steps, Vocational Rehabilitation Services, Medicaid and managed care areas.

ATTAIN GOAL: To increase the capacity of early childhood services to provide and pay for assistive technology devices and services on a statewide basis.

ATTAIN GOAL: To increase timely access of individuals with disabilities to assistive technology devices and services through department of education funding.

ATTAIN GOAL: To increase the timely access of persons with disabilities to assistive technology devices and services through vocational rehabilitation services.

ATTAIN GOAL: To increase timely access of persons with disabilities to alternative and augmentative communication devices and services funded through Medicaid.

ATTAIN GOAL: To assist in the development of policies, which allow for devices to transfer from funding sources as needed for customers needs.

ATTAIN GOAL: Increase the timely acquisition of durable medical equipment/assistive technology devices through private insurance policies.

ATTAIN GOAL: To increase the timely acquisition of wheeled mobility devices and services funded through Medicaid and Medicare.

ATTAIN GOAL: To monitor, review, and analyze managed care plans as they are being developed in regard to durable medical equipment/assistive technology devices and services.

ATTAIN GOAL: To increase the use of Plans to Achieve Self-Sufficiency to fund assistive technology devices and services.

Each of these goals was carefully chosen to match back to the mandated areas in the Tech Act, which are: Education, Vocational Rehabilitation, and medical assistance programs. The Tech Act states we must contract with Protection and Advocacy Services to assure systems change does occur. Protection and Advocacy stands ready to litigate if needed. To date, this aspect of the law has not been initiated. The SCT has been very successful in working collaboratively with the various state agencies involved to bring about incremental and on going changes.

Year Seven Systems Change Team (SCT) Outcomes

- **<u>Early Childhood:</u> Outcome on regulations, policies, attitudes, knowledge and skill level, practices and organizational structure. Total impact: 6,800 children with disabilities and 500 providers.**

⇒ Buy-Out Methodology for children with disabilities transitioning from First Steps to Part B Preschool programs. Assistive Technology (AT) devices that were used to reach developmental delay outcomes on the Individualized Family Service Plan (IFSP) and can also be used to meet the educational goals in the Individualized Education Plan (IEP). This "buy-out" provides a mechanism for Part B to purchase the device from First Steps and allows services to continue without delays of repurchasing the same device.

⇒ SCT worked with the First Steps task force to define "medical" versus "developmental delay" to determine who is responsible for the acquisition of AT for infants and toddlers with disabilities (OMPP, Children with Special Health Care Needs, CSHCN, or First Steps).

⇒ Assistive Technology for Infants and Toddlers: A transdisciplinary team assessment module that guides a team through the selection process of AT.

⇒ Submitted competencies to the IN Professional Standards Board for licensing requirements in AT for early childhood, general and special education teachers, and speech-language pathologist.

⇒ Worked with First Steps to develop a more precise tracking system when procuring AT devices at the local level.

- **<u>Education Part B:</u> Outcome on policies, knowledge and skill level, practices and organizational structure. Total impact: 117,000 students with disabilities and 66 special education planning districts.**

⇒ Define the circumstances under which case conference committees should consider recommending assessment of student's assistive technology needs.

⇒ Joint funding mechanism for assistive technology when a student is transitioning from school to adult services.

⇒ Work with Department of Education (DOE)/Division of Special Education (DSE) to develop guidelines for accommodations to be used during ISTEP test taking.

⇒ Work with DSE to develop a tracking system when AT devices are purchased at the local level.

- **Vocational Rehabilitation Services (VRS): Outcome on regulations, policies, attitudes, knowledge and skill level, practices, and organizational structure. Total impact: 41,300 consumers, 260 providers.**

⇒ "Buy-Out" Methodology: DDARS fiscal assisted DDARS/SCT through the Office of Budget Management to develop a cost formula of depreciation cost and address timeliness issue when student is transitioning from school to work. Vocational Rehabilitation is working with DSE to place the methodology in the "State Transition Plan Agreement" between VRS and DSE.

⇒ Develop a guideline for use by VR counselors defining the circumstances and intended purpose under which applicant's and clients AT needs are to be initially and periodically assessed.

⇒ Assistive Technology on the Job: A transdisciplinary team assessment module that guides a team through the selection process of AT.

⇒ Assure that rehabilitation technology services are provided consistent with the Rehab Act as amended in determining whether "comparable services" exist. SCT wrote to RSA requesting clarification of "What is Rehab Technology" and clarifying when it is exempt. VRS released an updated policy manual clarifying no comparable benefits search is required for rehabilitation technology services.

⇒ SCT is monitoring the new draft policy being developed for vehicle modifications. The SCT has given input in this process.

⇒ Identify and clarify situations where the Americans with Disabilities Act (ADA) or VRS is responsible for funding AT to students in post secondary. Information obtained from the AT Advocate has assisted in clarifying these situations and has been distributed to 57 disability services in post secondary schools and VRS.

- **Medicaid: Outcomes on regulations, policies, attitudes, knowledge and skill levels, practices, and organizational structure. Total Impact: 800,000 consumers and 14 providers and vendors of AAC devices.**

⇒ The SCT has reviewed the Medicaid state plan, policy and procedure codes on acquiring augmentative alternative communication devices through a task force of Medicaid and EDS personnel; the SCT, Speech-Language Pathologists, vendors of AAC devices, and an ATTAIN advisory board member. The Medicaid codes were changed from 2 generic codes to 6 specific codes for the AAC evaluation, purchase, rental, modification of the device, service (programming and training), and repair and maintenance.

⇒ Work with OMPP, EDS, providers and vendors to clarify and educate all parties about how to write "prior approvals and justifications" for purchase of AAC devices.

⇒ Work with OMPP and EDS to educate providers and vendors that physicians have the authority to sign off on prior approvals when an individual is enrolled in the Medicaid managed care program.

⇒ Work with providers, vendors, OMPP and EDS to resolve timely reimbursement of approved devices. Vendors are holding devices until they are reimbursed by OMPP, which adversely affects consumers.

⇒ Work with OMPP, EDS, and providers to develop a best practice guideline for acquisition of AAC devices and services.

- **Private Insurance and Managed Care: Outcome on laws, regulations, policies, attitudes, knowledge and skill level, practices and organizational structure. Total Impact: 800,000 consumers and 260 providers.**

⇒ Inconsistency in standard indemnity and managed care policies in the areas of grievance procedures, medical necessity and durable medical equipment.

⇒ SCT researched federal (including the Health Care Finance Administration, HCFA) and state guidelines on durable medical equipment, medical necessity and grievance procedures within private insurance, Medicare and Medicaid.

⇒ SCT worked with Department of Insurance to define durable medical equipment and medical necessity for the 1996 Legislative Session. These definitions were not introduced as legislation.

⇒ ATTAIN Co-Chairs the IN Task Force on Managed Care which introduced and passed HB 1663 providing timely resolution (an expedited 72 hours) of grievance procedures, giving information on access to services and a toll-free telephone number to file a grievance procedure.

⇒ IN Task Force on Managed Care working with the Department of Insurance to develop the regulations and a "report card" for consumers to compare indemnity or managed care insurance policies.

⇒ IN Task Force on Managed Care held first conference to educate consumers and decision makers about the impact of managed care on individuals with disabilities. Approximately 220 people attended.

⇒ IN Task Force on Managed Care developed an educational brochure about the "ABC"s of Choosing a Managed Care Plan"

⇒ IN Task Force on Managed Care worked with OMPP and others to design a Medicaid managed care program for individuals with chronic health care needs.

- **Medicaid/Medicare timely acquisition of wheeled mobility: Outcome on policies, knowledge and skill level, and practices. Total Impact: 139,200 consumers and 17 providers.**

⇒ SCT reviewed IAC code to define the term "customized wheelchair" (fabricated from the ground up) versus "standard" wheelchairs that could have customized seating. Standard wheelchairs are included in the daily per diem.

⇒ SCT discussed and resolved 7 cases.

⇒ Medicare beneficiaries don't understand the difference between providers who accept "assignment and nonassignment"

- **To increase the use of Plans to Achieve Self Sufficiency (PASS) through Social Security to fund assistive technology devices and services. Outcome on knowledge and skill level, and practices. Total Impact 60,000 consumers and 500 providers.**

⇒ Educate and inform individuals how to utilize PASS plans as a funding source for assistive technology.

⇒ Monitor federal changes in Social Security regarding PASS and share with individuals at the ATTAIN Funding Conference in May of 1998 and through the Empowerment and Advocacy Training's held four times yearly.

OTHER FEDERAL/ATTAIN PRIORITY OUTCOMES

FEDERAL/ATTAIN PRIORITY ONE:

- ATTAIN has introduced an Assistive Technology Consumer Protection Bill for the past three years. The bill requires manufacturers of defective devices to provide a 90 day to one year warranty on assistive devices purchased by state agencies or individuals with disabilities. It also provides a mechanism for repair or replacement after the device has been repaired twice. HB 1332 made it out of the committee but died on second reading.
- Action alerts were sent to more than 500 individuals on the ATTAIN advisory board, empowerment and advocacy and community technology networks. Action Alert topics were: Reauthorization of IDEA, ISTEP Plus testing, regulations on the Rehab Act, managed care and the AT Consumer Protection Bill.
- Other activities were included in the systems change outcomes.

FEDERAL/ATTAIN PRIORITY TWO:

- Over the past seven and one half years, ATTAIN has produced several modules to educate and train consumers and service providers about various aspects of AT. Those modules are: *Accessibility, Accommodation and Assistive Technology: A Guidebook to Empowering Individuals with Disabilities; Indiana Resources: Assistive Technology Funding Guide* (this module is in it's first revision); *Best Practice Guideline for AAC*; four (4) modules for Transdisciplinary team AT assessments: *Assistive Technology for Infants and Toddlers, Assistive Technology for Education, Assistive Technology on the Job, and Assistive Technology for Persons who are Elderly;* twelve (12) *Assistive Technology Higher Education* modules to train pre-service students in the area of AT.
- Breaking New Ground has developed a *Caregivers* module with contributing funds from ATTAIN.
- Other activities were included in the systems change outcomes.

FEDERAL/ATTAIN PRIORITY THREE:

- These activities were included in the systems change outcomes.

FEDERAL/ATTAIN PRIORITY FOUR:

- ATTAIN hosted four Empowerment and Advocacy Trainings which impacted 671 consumers and service providers from rural and urban areas of the state.
- ATTAIN Empowerment and Advocacy graduates provide training and systems change in their local communities. Some of those changes have included: attendance at public hearings like VRS' 3 year state plan, training parent groups on accessing AT and services, transition, education, early intervention and accommodations and accessibility issues such as curb cuts and renovation to local libraries.
- Working with Minority Health Care Coalitions to identify services which resulted in the *ATTAIN Directory of Resources*
- Other activities were included in the systems change outcomes.

FEDERAL/ATTAIN PRIORITY FIVE:

- Outreach activities occurred at National Vision Rehabilitation Day Expo, transition and community health fairs, Black Expo, Aging Conference, IN Deaf Heritage Days, "Brag and Steal Meetings", businesses, Independent Living Centers and state and local agencies. Impact 4,923 consumers and service providers.
- Community Technology Networks (CTN): These networks identify barriers that impede the availability of AT in their local communities and problem solve on possible solutions. 321 consumers and service providers participate in these CTN's statewide.
- Other activities were included in the systems change outcome.

FEDERAL/ATTAIN PRIORITY SIX:

- Timely acquisition for AT is occurring through 223 individual advocacy cases involving Medicaid, education, Medicare, Vocational Rehabilitation, and the Department of Insurance.
- A CTN and 2 libraries wrote Department of Commerce and received $140,000 to pay for accessible computer equipment and the training to use the computers.
- Another CTN worked with local agencies to lend AT back and forth among the agencies to benefit consumers.
- ATTAIN developed a directory of organizations that provide assessments: *Indiana Assessment Resource Guide.*
- The Assistive Technology Higher Education Consortium has been instrumental in assisting universities in developing basic courses such as "Fundamental of AT"; Vincennes University has established an AT Certificate Program and is working to obtain approval from the IN Higher Education Commission to establish an associate degree program in AT.
- ATTAIN's Equipment Exchange Network is a medium that allows consumers to buy, sell, loan or give away AT. The Exchange has 255 listings and growing.
- ATTAIN is set aside $150,000 to establish an Alternative Loan Program for consumers who are not eligible for state programs.
- ATTAIN has set aside $175,000 to establish Assistive Technology Demonstration and Loan Sites to assist consumers in obtaining transdisciplinary assessments, and a place to try or borrow AT to assure the device is most appropriate.

ATTAIN ANNUAL STATISTICAL REPORT

YEAR	I&R	TRNG.	OUTREACH DISSEM.	TECH.ASS'T. ASSISTANCE	INDIV. CASE ADVOCACY
1991	not avail.	not avail.	not avail.	not avail.	
1992	not avail.	not avail.	10,000	not avail.	
1993	2,799	1,449	27,517	1,081	
1994	1,303	2,848	27,040	28	
1995	2,786	594	7,500	1,474	
1996	2,784	12,690	7,098	48	??
1997	2,789	2,269	4,874	720	223
TOTAL	**12,461**	**19,850**	**74,029**	**3,581**	

- After March 1994, Tech Act Projects were mandated to provide individual case advocacy. States had one year to transition. 1995-1996 ATTAIN began educating consumers about these services.
- 1995 was the first year Tech Act Projects began to use the NIDRR reporting form. Therefore, there is some inconsistency in which data was reported.
- In 1996 the forms indicated staff mixed the areas of technical assistance and training. Their goal was no duplicated numbers.
- Note: As project shifted focus on systemic change, numbers changed accordingly.

Buy-Out Methodology

In those instances where a student has been provided an assistive technology device by the local education agency (LEA) and the student is ready to transition from school to adult programming through Vocational Rehabilitation Services (VRS), VRS and the client determine if the assistive technology device will continue to adequately meet the needs of the individual in VR sponsored training or in employment. If the LEA does not wish to retain the device for assignment to another student, the VR counselor may wish to consider proposing to purchase the device from the LEA. The following would be the recommended approach to be utilized in making such an AT buy-out proposal:

(Note: Research in federal regulations as to equipment depreciation by DDARS has revealed that Education Regulations (EDGAR) are not specific and as a result, the depreciation strategy defined in OMB Circular A-87 should be utilized to determine the current value of used equipment.)

The following procedure is based on OMB Circular A-87's method of depreciating equipment (computers and other types of equipment.)

If the LEA is willing to consider possibility of sale to VR:

1. VR Counselor obtains a copy of original purchase invoice from LEA.
2. VR Counselor calculates current value of used equipment.
   a. Computers are regarded to have a useful life expectancy of 5 years. Other types of equipment are regarded as having 7 years useful life expectancy. AAC devices utilizing computer technology have 5 years useful life expectancy.
   b. Prorate value based on original purchase cost, age, and remaining useful life of equipment.

For example, for a 3 year old augmentative communication device, whose original purchase cost was $5,000...

1) Calculate depreciation
   Age of equipment (A) divided by life expectancy of equipment LE times purchase cost (PC) equals depreciation (D)
   (A/LE)xPC=D
   (3years/5years) x $5,000 = $3,000 depreciation
2) Find current value
   Original purchase cost (OPC) minus depreciation (D) equals current value (CV)
   OPC - D = CV
   $5,000 - $3,000 = $2,000

- In determining age of equipment it is permissible to round off to the nearest year.

As a device reaches near the end of it's useful life expectancy, more consideration should be given to the purchase of new assistive technology as opposed to buying out the older equipment.

If the original cost included mounting (as to a wheelchair) or adaptation costs, these are appropriate to include in the original cost/figure, if such mounting or adaptation will continue to be needed for the individual to utilize the device in their adult program.

The cost of initial training or programming of the device should not be included in the original cost figure as this should deal only with the actual equipment cost.

3. VR counselor makes a written proposal to appropriate LEA officials, specifying the proposed purchase price (current value) and showing the detail/rational from step two used in arriving at the proposed purchase price.

4. LEA either accepts or denies the proposed buy-out in writing. If accepted the purchase proceeds according to standard VR authorization/claim voucher process. If denied by the LEA , VR and client plan to meet the individual's AT need by purchasing new devices/services.

5. If the LEA does accept the proposal, once the LEA has received payment for the device, a receipt should be issued by the LEA to VRS with title/papers, warranty if any, ownership papers, operators manual, etc., to be provided to the client, consistent with VRS policy.

6. As with any other equipment purchase by VRS, VRS retains title to the equipment until such time at successful closure when title may be transferred to the client, consistent with VRS policy.

- Although several Vocational Rehabilitation offices and Local Education Agencies have adopted this Buy-Out Methodology, there is no formal agreement at this time between Educational and Vocational Rehabilitation Services or between Early Intervention Services and Education.

This handout speaks of transition from Education to Vocational Rehabilitation Services. The same method may be used in transition from Early Intervention Services to Education.

Assistive Technology
A One-Year Program Leading to A Certificate of Program Completion

Major Course -- Departmental Requirements		*Credit Hours*
APS 251	Fundamentals of Assistive Technology	3
APS 261	Assessment, Selection, and Evaluation of AT	3
APS 265	Funding and Policy Issues in Assistive Technology	3
APS 271	Applications in Assistive Technology	3
APS 275	Internship/Special Project in Assistive Technology	3

Major Course -- Program Requirements

APS 142	General Psychology or Applied Psychology	3
APS 291	Introduction to Exceptionalities or equivalent	3
AED 200	Computers in the Classroom (Preferred) or Computers for Technology	2-3

English Composition Requirement

HEW 101	English Composition I	3

Optional:

APS 279	Review Course for Assistive Technology Credentialing	1

Assistive Technology
A Two-Year Program Leading to the A.A.S. Degree

Major Course-Departmental Requirements

APS 251	Fundamentals of Assistive Technology	3
APS 261	Assessment, Selection, and Evaluation of AT	3
APS 265	Funding and Policy Issues in Assistive Technology	3
APS 271	Applications in Assistive Technology	3
APS 275	Internship/Special Project in Assistive Technology	3

Major Courses-Program Requirements

AGS 100	Introduction to Social Sciences	1
APS 142	General Psychology	3
APS 201	Developmental Psychology or Psychology of Growth and Change	3
APS 291	Introduction to Exceptionalities	3
ASO 151	Principles of Sociology	3
SLS/SLL 111	Anatomy and Physiology I or Laboratory Science	3-4
HSS 141/143	Interpersonal Communication or or Speech equivalent	2 - 3
DHR 110	Medical Terminology for Allied Health	3
AED 200	Computers in the Classroom or Computers for Technology	2-3
PPR 249	Recreation and Special Populations	3

English Composition Requirement

HEW 101	English Composition I	3
HEW 102	English Composition II	3

Physical Education Activity Requirement

Two PE Activity Courses (PPF & PPE) or First Aid		2
Mathematics Elective (SMA 100 or higher)		3
Humanities Elective		3
*Electives		9
Optional		
APS 279	Review Course for Assistive Technology Credentialing	0-1
		64-67

***Recommended Electives:** Community Rehabilitation I, Ethics in the Helping Professions, Courses required for related disciplines.*

ATTAIN'S MISSION

All

People

With

Disabilities

In Indiana

Will

Have Access To

Assistive

Technology.

You may contact us at our
E-mail address:
CFulford@vunet.vinu.edu

ATTAIN is federally funded through the Technology Related Assistance for Individuals With Disabilities Act Amendments of 1994, Public Law 103-218. Indiana Division of Disability, Aging and Rehabilitative Services is the lead agency for the project.

The **Empowerment and Advocacy Training Network** is a three day workshop designed for individuals with disabilities, family members and authorized representatives. The training/workshop instructs each "trainer" on the laws, regulations, policies, practices and procedures in regard to accessing assistive technology devices and services and effective strategies for obtaining assistive technology. The "trainers" are placed on the Empowerment and Advocacy Network through which customers, family members and interested others can link up for knowledge.

The **Equipment Exchange Network** (EEN) is available to assist any individual interested in the sale, purchase, trade, loan or donation of assistive technology devices. The EEN surveys customers, organizations and agencies who have assistive technology devices not currently in use to place on the network. The EEN is available through the ATTAIN Newsletter (quarterly publication) or by calling the central office.

ATTAIN Outreach Affiliations

Through travel in a mobile van to rural and underserved communities, the **Breaking New Ground Rural Outreach Program** provides public awareness, demonstration and technical assistance regarding the potential applications of assistive technology and modifications to agricultural equipment, worksites and homes to improve the quality of life of rural residents and farmers with disabilities in Indiana.

Breaking New Ground
Purdue University
1146 Agricultural Engineer Building
West Lafayette, IN 47907-1146
(800) 825-4264
(765) 494-5088–Voice/TT

The **Assistive Technology Higher Education Consortium** (ATHE), Vincennes University, provides a structure of representatives that will study the current level of assistive technology instruction in Indiana. More information is available by calling the central office.

The **Assistive Technology, Training and Information Center** (ATTIC) is an alliance for technology access site designed to empower individuals with special needs and their families to access services and activities, from a range of acceptable options, which lead to the greatest level of independence. ATTIC provides technical assistance for assistive technology, equipment demonstration, and public awareness about issues regarding assistive technology for individuals with disabilities.

ATTIC
3354 Pine Hill Drive
Vincennes, IN 47591
(800) 962-8842
(812) 886-0575

The purpose of the ATTAIN Project is to create systems change by developing a comprehensive, customer responsive statewide program. The project promotes community based, technology related services through training and outreach activities, empowerment and advocacy activities, individual case advocacy on funding issues, policy review, and position statements.

What Is Assistive Technology?

Assistive technology is "any item, piece of equipment or product system, whether acquired commercially off the shelf, modified or customized, that is used to increase, maintain or improve functional capabilities of individuals with disabilities." Examples of assistive technology include modified computer input and output such as adapted keyboards, braille and large print, mobility aids such as walkers and wheelchairs; augmentative and alternative communication aids, environmental control systems such as automatic lighting or alarm systems; recreational aids or adapted toys and home/worksite modifications such as ramps or grab bars.

Many services which relate to technology and its use by individuals with disabilities are offered through the ATTAIN Project. General information about ATTAIN and statewide technology related assistance services is available toll-free by calling the central office.

Through empowerment and case advocacy, the ATTAIN Systems Change Team Coordinators (**Adult Services, Education, and Medical Assistance Coordinators**) work with individuals who have difficulty accessing assistive technology devices and services in education, medical programs and adult services.

The ATTAIN **Training Coordinator** coordinates all ATTAIN trainings, demonstrations, and workshops including collaboration with training components from our three program areas. ATTAIN utilizes a Staff and Community Training Network to meet disability related, topic specific training needs.

The ATTAIN **Community Consultants** work with local communities to develop and facilitate the use of assistive technology in all areas of life. Customers, providers, employers, and the general public make up the local Community Technology Networks.

A **Community Technology Network** (CTN) is an informal gathering of people who identify barriers that occur when an individual with a disability attempts to access assistive technology in their community. The CTN develops a plan of action to resolve the identified barriers. Barriers

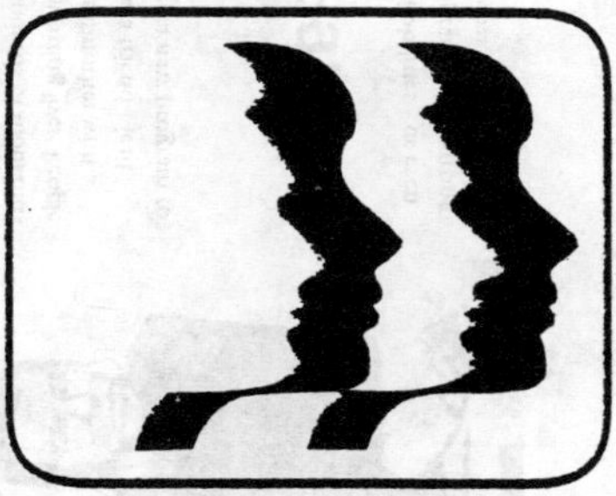

may involve state and local laws, policies and practices and procedures. The CTNS are empowered to make a difference in local communities. Participants are encouraged to complete ATTAIN's Empowerment and Advocacy Training offered each year. Members receive "Action Alerts" regarding legislation that impacts disability issues.

ATTAIN — Increased Independence — Accessing Technology Through Awareness in Indiana

ATTAIN
Central Office

1815 N. Meridian Street
Suite 200
Indianapolis, IN 46202

(317) 921-8766
(317) 921-8774-FAX

(800) 5·A·T·T·A·I·N
Toll Free
(In Indiana)

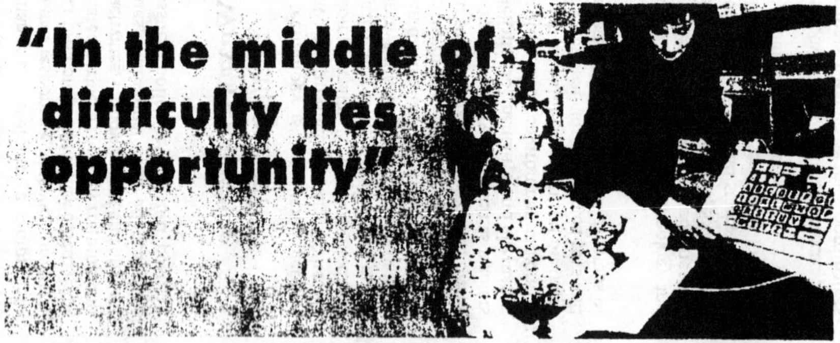

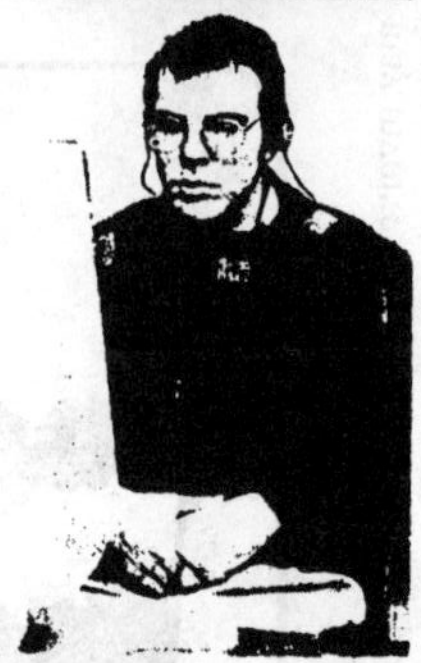

Thanks to technology - and the professionals adapting its use - hundreds of thousands of people with disabilities are beginning to live more productive, rewarding lives. People like the little girl in home-room who has cerebral palsy or the grandmother with a broken hip. Today technology can help you - as a professional and a friend - lead people to a better way of life. And Vincennes University is offering a new program to show you how.

It's called Assistive Technology.

You don't necessarily have to work exclusively with people with disabilities - or even have any prior experience in technology - to benefit from this program. Just a strong desire to learn some new skills so you can work smarter with fresh ideas and techniques,

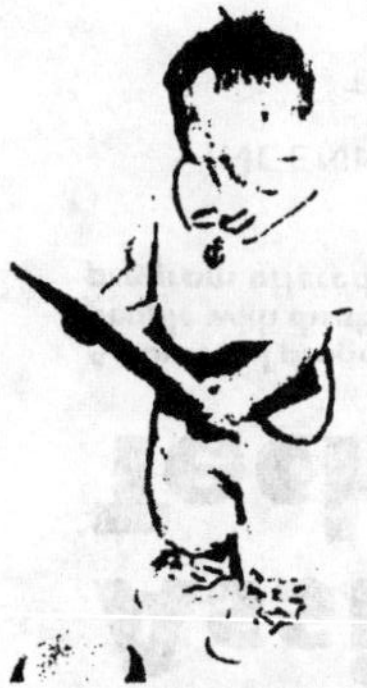

Technology is improving quality of life . . .

- Smart mechanical devices can compensate for nerves or muscles that no longer respond
- Computer modifications and sophisticated software have enhanced productivity, functioning and learning
- Electronics can translate speech to the written word or the written word to speech.
- Adapted toys and recreational supplies have made it possible for children of all ages to pla independently.
- Improvements in orthopedic and prosthetic devices have brought vast improvements in mobility, independence, and career opportunities for people with disabilities.
- Simple, low-cost devices can help individuals participate in the mainstream of society at home, school, work, and in the community.

Who should enroll?

- Students or professionals who desire a rewarding career and want to learn more about the impact of technology on the lives of people with disabilities at home, school, work, and in the community.
- Students who are pursuing degrees in general education, special education, psychology, rehabilitation, behavioral sciences, sociology, gerontology, social work, occupational therapy, physical therapy, nursing, architecture, engineering, business, or any disability-related curriculum and want to specialize in assistive technology.
- Students or professionals who are interested in learning about available assistive devices and services that can benefit people with disabilities

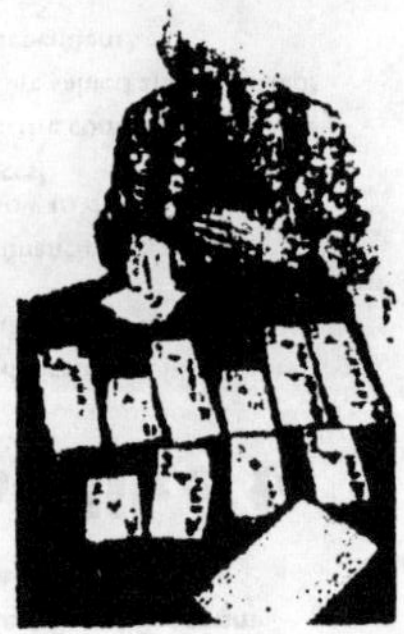

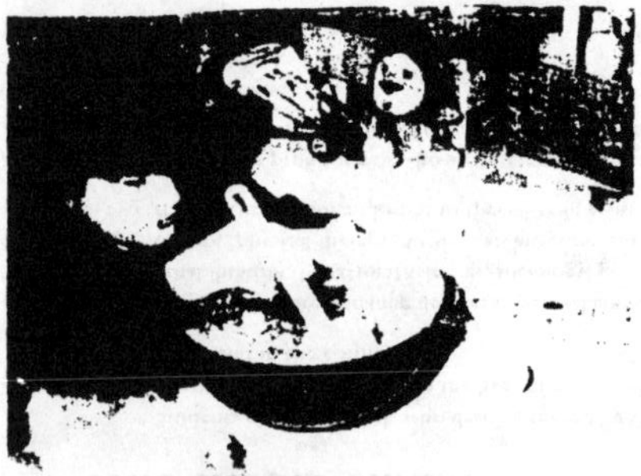

The Assistive Technology Certificate Program
will help you professionally.

Wouldn't you like to

- Enhance your career track?
- Increase your confidence as an advocate and instructor?
- Have a better understanding of the trends and issues surrounding this field?
- Learn about successful, creative financing strategies?
- Have access to information on how to design and deliver quality assistive technology services?
- Recognize the components of effective community services?
- Share in a vision where all people are valued and respected?
- Empower people to be more independent?

Assistive Technology

A powerful program for anyone interested in helping people with disabilities gain independence. Certificate program offered exclusively in Indiana by

VINCENNES UNIVERSITY
The Two-Year College

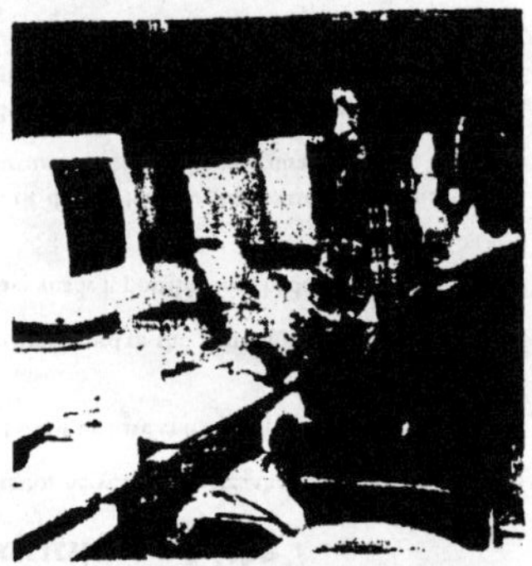

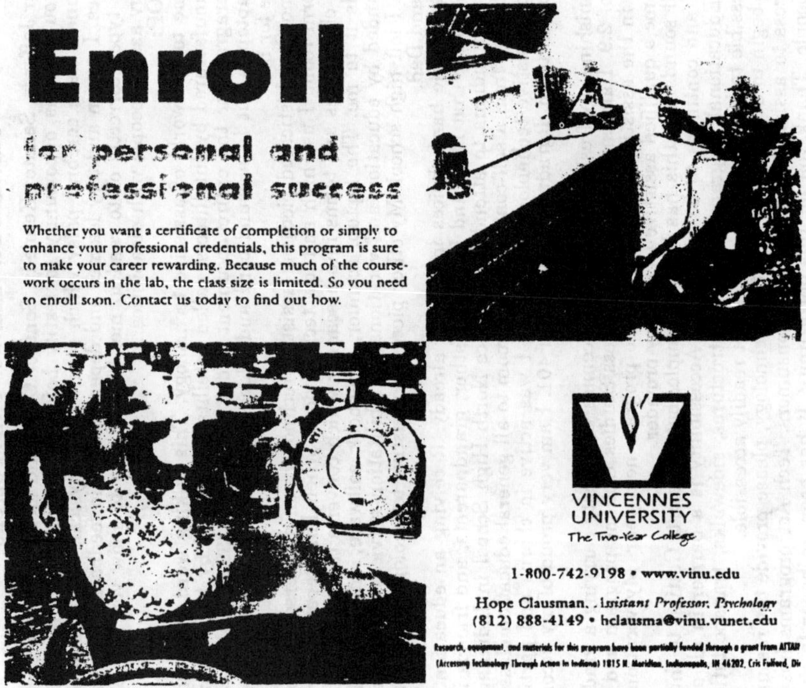
Enroll
for personal and professional success
Whether you want a certificate of completion or simply to enhance your professional credentials, this program is sure to make your career rewarding. Because much of the coursework occurs in the lab, the class size is limited. So you need to enroll soon. Contact us today to find out how.
VINCENNES UNIVERSITY
The Two-Year College
1-800-742-9198 • www.vinu.edu
Hope Clausman, Assistant Professor, Psychology
(812) 888-4149 • hclausma@vinu.vunet.edu
Research, equipment, and materials for this program have been partially funded through a grant from ATTAIN
(Accessing Technology Through Action in Indiana) 1815 N. Meridian, Indianapolis, IN 46202, Cris Fulford, Dir

PREPARED STATEMENT OF CRAIG FULFORD

Senator Jeffords, Senator Kennedy, Senator Coats and members of the committee: Thank you for this opportunity to testify before you today. My name is Craig Fulford and I have cerebral palsy which resulted in physical, visual, and learning disabilities. I am an auditory learner and depend on audio feedback to let me know if I have typed correctly or to read to me. I would like to show you how assistive technology assists people with disabilities.

LAPTOP:

Welcome to the world of assistive technology. This talking word processing program manufactured by Intellitools, called Intellitalk will read by letter, word, sentence, paragraph or the entire document and it only costs $39.95. All we've done to this laptop is put in a sound card and added a software program to make this accessible for me.

I use more sophisticated pieces of assistive technology on my personnel computer in my dorm room. I use high and low tech devices. When I'm preparing for a test, I scan in class notes and terms into a scanner which converts the material to Word and reads it to me. The laptop, scanner, Openbook software, and Dec talk were jointly funded by education and vocational rehabilitation services and exited with me when I left high school. My other pieces of assistive technology were purchased by Mom and Dad.

I've made some hard choices in my life already. Receiving an education was so important to me that Mom and I left my father, grandparents, and friends in rural southwestern Indiana to attend L Lawrence North High School in Indianapolis. It was hard to go from a self-contained classroom to all general education classes with the use of assistive technology. But I did. I was active in chorus and participated on the speech team. I graduated 138 out of 401. I am very proud of my accomplishments.

I am finishing my freshman year at Vincennes University carrying a grade point average of 2.9. I am enrolled in the Business Studies Options program and will be enrolling in the assistive technology degree program next year. My vocational goal is to become a qualified assistive technology provider.

This all sounds like this has been so simple, but it hasn't. Getting to this point has been and continues to be a struggle. Accessibility is a barrier in all areas of my life. Educational programs, building structures, sidewalks, transportation and even accessible technology is doable, but not readily accessible.

As you begin to decide about assistive technology, please provide the resources for direct access to assistive technology for consumers. Tech Act programs has helped a lot of people. Thank you for this opportunity. It has been an honor to share my assistive technology and thoughts.

AUTOBIOGRAPHY OF CRAIG FULFORD

Craig Fulford is a twenty-two year old student enrolled in the Business Studies Options program at Vincennes University. Craig was born with cerebral palsy resulting in a physical, visual and learning disabilities. He is an extensive user of assistive technology both low and high technology devices.

Craig has become a trainer in the ATTAIN Empowerment and Advocacy program working with local communities to infuse assistive technology. He has provided demonstrations and presentations on the various assistive technology devices he uses at national, state and local conferences and trainings. He has also participated in the summer session of Partners in Policymaking.

In 1989 Craig testified in the Indiana Senate on behalf of House Bill 1789, "Transition for Youth with Disabilities". In 1994 Craig testified in the Indiana General Assembly House Ways and Means Committee about allowing schools to purchase assistive technology for students with disabilities in the State Technology Plan Grants.

Because the quality of Craig's education is so important to him, he and his family have challenged the educational system to be included in general education settings using assistive technology.

This past and upcoming summer, Craig works half days in a radio station and attends the university summer sessions. He also volunteers as a peer advocate with other high school students with disabilities.

The CHAIRMAN. Thank you. that was a very, very strong and helpful statement.

Craig, you are to be commended for volunteering to work with high school students with disabilities. What kinds of questions do they ask you about technology, and how do you help them?

Mr. FULFORD. Basically, they ask me where they can go to get this technology, and I go about leading them mostly in another direction. She is the best one to get them started, and then, if she does not know the way, she can guide them in other directions.

The CHAIRMAN. Thank you.

Before I continue, I want to remind everyone about the expo this afternoon. It is from 2 to 4, and it is on the ground floor of the Dirksen Building in Room G-50. There are 26 assistive technology exhibits there, and I hope you will all have a chance to attend.

I have many other questions, but unfortunately, we have run out of time by more than an hour. I would like to get some thoughts on what we should do in regard to the 10-year cycle. For the tech projects that have not received 10 years of Federal funding, we intend to ensure that the 10-year cycle does not impede the flexibility and creativity in addressing assistive technology needs in a particular State.

However, are there certain accomplishments that we can expect from each State as it moves toward the end of a 10-year cycle of Federal funding?

Ms. Cleveland.

Ms. CLEVELAND. I think it is reasonable to expect that, as each State finishes out its 10-year cycle, they have made efforts, as was the direction of the Tech Act, to create some sustainability within systems, whether they make their demo and trial centers sustainable, whether they find sustainable funding sources for various activities. I think it is reasonable to expect that that will happen in every State.

However, I think that beyond the 10 years, there remains a need for some of the core activities that all the State Tech Act projects do, such as the systems policy work that we do, the training efforts that are ongoing, and also the ability to meet the new challenges as they arise, as technology changes, as information technology becomes a greater issue and access issues remain, that it will be important for Tech Act projects or State to have the ability to meet those needs.

The CHAIRMAN. Any other comments?

Mr. PAWLEK. I would just echo Lynne's comments. Again, I would look at it a little bit from the marketplace point of view, realizing that some of the things that we do, because of what they do, will be absorbed easily and quickly, or somewhat quickly, into the systems. There will be support for those things. For other things, there is a lot more difficulty getting support.

Part of our job is in fact marketing technology, and the more we do that, the more need there is, so we get into a bit of a vicious cycle, but it is a good cycle, really, assuming we can continue to meet those needs.

The CHAIRMAN. How long have you been with the New Hampshire Project?

Mr. PAWLEK. Seven years.

The CHAIRMAN. Have you seen a lot of changes?

Mr. PAWLEK. A huge amount of changes certainly from when I started, which was the original Tech Act, to where things are now. I think there is much more awareness around technology as an issue, but again, still many questions and many issues to be resolved with the changes in managed care—things that we have talked about here—the demographics of the aging population, the internet. It is just vast different.

The CHAIRMAN. Ms. Fulford?

Ms. Fulford. I would reiterate what I said in my testimony, that information is important, yes, because until you have a need to know, you do not bother to find out about assistive technology. So that is going to be an ongoing need.

Systems change and working with the systems to make them coordinate together for assistive technology funding is very important, but also, the training piece is a piece that must continue to be in there, to educate and train not only consumers but service providers, because one thing we found when we began our empowerment and advocacy training, which we are well-known for, was that we had consumers knowing more than service providers, and service providers were coming back to us and asking, could we please sit at the table and hear the same thing. It was a really unique experience, and now we do it through a team method of training. They have to bring together teams to this training. So that was unique.

Those are three integral pieces, and I think that adding State flexibility, because what works for Lynne does not work for me. Each State is unique, with its own different characteristics, and the way one State can handle it, I may not be able to handle it that way. So I think that that is an important component that needs to be continued.

The CHAIRMAN. Ms. Cleveland, you have the last word.

Ms. CLEVELAND. I would definitely echo the absolute need for State flexibility in whatever future assistive technology legislation is passed, because as Cris has just said, we have 56 very unique entities out there that learn from each other and have done a lot in terms of not duplicating efforts but also need to be able to do original things that work just for them.

The CHAIRMAN. Thank you all so much for very helpful testimony. I appreciate the work you are doing out there where it really counts, and we will be in touch with you, and hopefully, if we need some help, you will be there for us.

Thank you very much. All members will have the right to put statements in the record.

With that, we will close the hearing.

[Whereupon, at 1:08 p.m., the committee was adjourned.]

○

APEX
TP
9780160571589
76901945–76